PRAISE FOR THE 100 YEAR LIFESTYLE

"Dr. Plasker has committed many years to developing health and wellness programs for communities around the country. His book reflects this same commitment and will help you improve the quality of your life."

Stedman Graham, founder of Athletes Against Drugs

"Dr. Plasker's innovative *100 Year Lifestyle Fitness Assessment* on getting your ESS in Shape – your endurance, strength, and structure – will help you add years to your life and quality of life to your years."

Scott Goudeseune, President, American Council on Exercise

"Dr. Plasker's care and *The 100 Year Lifestyle* concepts have helped me greatly improve my competitiveness and I am certain will ultimately extend my athletic career. I have always put a great deal of stress on my spine and skeletal structure, especially while training for the world record modified bench press, and with the help of Dr. Plasker's care I was able to set the World Record of 360 pounds. You need this in your life!"

Kyle Maynard, world record holder and bestselling author of *No Excuses*

"Dr. Plasker reveals the time-tested principles to living your best life in this easy-to-read guide that makes living well a reality for all. Read this book and discover how to dramatically increase both the quality and the quantity of your years."

Dr. Bob Hoffman, CEO of Masters Circle

"Dr. Plasker's principles make living to 100 exciting, rather than frightening. You will benefit from these life changing health, relationship, and financial principles today, tomorrow, and every day for the rest of your life."

Ivan Misner, Ph.D., founder of BNI and New York Times bestselling author

"Dr. Plasker has created the opportunity for people to live the health of their dreams at every age. This book is fun to read, very practical, and easy to follow. I really appreciate the reflective points and self-responsibility it promotes. Well done. Again, an ounce of prevention is worth a pound of cure."

Dr. Liz Anderson-Peacock, CEO, Girls, Gals and Gurus, Inc., a healthy lifestyle company for women

"In *The 100 Year Lifestyle*, Dr. Plasker addresses a marvelous question that our over-stressed society must think about, 'What if I were to live to 100?' As this book points out, the implications are huge. In the chaotic world of wellness, this book stands out as unique, powerful, and immensely practical…not to mention, it is a lot of fun. Read this and learn to live well, to 100 and beyond."

Dr. Patrick Gentempo, Jr., CEO, Creating Wellness, Inc.

"I applaud the guidelines set forth in Dr. Plasker's book, *The 100 Year Lifestyle*."

Jack LaLanne

ADDITIONAL PRAISE FOR THE 100 YEAR LIFESTYLE 2ND EDITION

"In my journey to re-establish my own health after being diagnosed with thyroid cancer, The 100 Year Lifestyle principles helped me get my health back, and inspired me to help others to make changes in their lifestyle, including Chiropractic care, so that they could live their best life every day!"

Dr. Amber Eckel

"*The 100 Year Lifestyle* has been a life-changing catalyst for me to lose 375 pounds and find the life I never knew I could have."

Terry Chaney, Chiropractic Assistant

"People spend their entire lives striving for health and wealth. *The 100 Year Lifestyle* shows you how to have it now and sustain it for a lifetime. This book will make you healthy, wealthy and wise."

Garrett Gunderson, NY Times Bestselling Author, *Killing Sacred Cows*

"The *100 Year Lifestyle* is the plan of action for you to turn your health care and life paradigm around. Life University is proud to be associated with this profound concept and movement."

Dr. Guy Riekeman, President, Life University

"*The 100 Year Lifestyle* principles are right on. Dr. Plasker defines a new health care and lifestyle model for you and your family to live by, and it is good for the world. I taught it in New Zealand for years and will continue to share this important message with individuals and leaders here in the States. *The 100 Year Lifestyle* is an idea whose time has come."

Dr. Brian Kelly, President, Life Chiropractic College West

"So if you haven't read Dr. Plasker's first book then all I can say is you missed out and there is never a better time to get up to speed on what living *The 100 Year Lifestyle* is all about. I personally have found that Dr. Plasker's insights are practical and as a health professional they are the GOLD standard for helping others take back their health and life. As the President of the California Chiropractic Association it is my mission to get information that can support health to our patients in every office and this latest book will be the vehicle I will use to help assist in turning America's health crisis around."

Dr. Matt Hubbard, President California Chiropractic Association

"A true visionary, Dr. Plasker's *The 100 Year Lifestyle* enlightens us on how to achieve our greatest human potential. The ONE Concept Community embraces and lives this vision. It is time for us all to do the same. Let this vision guide you to the healthy, happy, fulfilling life you deserve."

Monica Pasinato-Forchielli B.Comm, RMT, founder & Chief Visionary Officer ONE Concept

"Health Care is in need of an overhaul and there are so many people who need to adjust their lifestyle. In *The 100 Year Lifestyle*, Dr. Plasker provides an Innate philosophy and strategy that every man, woman, and child, can live by to optimize their health and function at their full God given potential."

Dr. Edwin Cordero, President, Sherman College of Chiropractic

"I have known Dr. Plasker for more than 15 years as a teacher, mentor and friend. He is a master communicator and his books make it so easy for his readers to take action, make changes and live the life they were meant to live. This book is not only a game changer, it is a life changer!"

Dr. Brian Stenzler, Vice President California Chiropractic Association

"*The 100 Year Lifestyle* transcends the typical and often confusing world of prevention and wellness, by inspiring the reader to find their personal "why" as it relates to their life goals, and then gives them the simple, yet profound tools for creating a lifestyle that maximizes their potential...physically, mentally, spiritually, socially and financially."

Dr. John Bueler, Jr., Past President California Chiropractic Association

"Dr. Plasker has given the world an incredible message. This creates a tremendous opportunity and responsibility for health care providers to help people realize their potential rather than wait for a crisis. For our culture, this can transform the health of humanity. *The 100 Year Lifestyle* is more than a book; it is a mindset and attitude that can help you feel great every day on your way to 100 years and beyond!"

Dr. Dennis R. Buckley, Author *The Hole In Your Diploma, What You Forgot To Learn In Chiropractic College* and *S.C.O.R.E. Student Chiropractors On Road To Excellence*

"Dr. Plasker's *The 100 Year Lifestyle 2nd Edition*, has captured some of the most relevant and important information regarding something that affects us all...longevity. Living a long life is one thing. Living a long, quality life is something completely different. The valuable information contained in this book has transformed our practice and the community we serve. This is a must read for all who look forward to living a long and vibrant life."

Dr. Jack Bourla

"Through our practice and online women's community, Educated Pregnancy, we have been empowering millions of families with the tools they need to make healthy lifestyle choices. By sharing *The 100 Year Lifestyle*, we are able to effectively reach more people on a grander scale to truly impact the lives of generations to come."

Dr. Cathy Wendland-Colby and Dr. Norm Colby

"Since its first publication, *The 100 Year Lifestyle* has become "the text book" for living life to the fullest. I have seen the principles and concepts in this book literally change the lives of thousands of people in our community. This book is a "life changer" for anyone, at any age, who is interested in living their full expression of life."

Dr. David Moore, Chiropractor and author of *The Chiropractic Evolution*

"I have known Dr. Plasker for more than a decade and he is an extremely purposeful and committed individual. *The 100 Year Lifestyle* will teach you, in very simple and practical ways, to express your full potential and experience the power of self-healing for a lifetime."

Dr. Fabrizio Mancini, bestselling author *The Power of Self-Healing*

"I've helped thousands of patients over the years with many conditions, chronic pain and degeneration of the spine. You don't have to age that way. The good news is that you have the solution in your hands to living an active, healthy, long life. Enjoy it!"

Dr. Aixa Goodrich

"Few doctors in the world exhibit the passion and purpose of Dr. Eric Plasker to make a real difference in the quality of people's lives and the world. In his new book the "change master" will share with you strategies and lifestyle choices that will allow you to better express your innate potential. Dr. Plasker will inspire you with this uncommonly common sense plan to regain your life and set you on track to living full out. Jump on board *The 100 Year Lifestyle* train and leave the unsustainable, reactionary, disease care model of crazy town behind once and for all. Welcome to the brave new world of optimized living!"

Dr. Liam P. Schubel

"I have known Dr. Plasker for 30 years and have found him to be a principled man, husband, father and chiropractor who is committed to changing the world one person and community at a time. Through The 100 Year Lifestyle 2nd Edition, he delivers an Innate philosophy that is simple and easy for people to understand. Practice and live these principles and you are sure to live up to your Innate potential throughout your lifetime."

Dr. DD Humber, FICA, Past President International Chiropractors Association

"Many have put out information on healthy living but Dr. Plasker is the first to put it all together with the multiple components necessary to assure good health and a meaningful life from birth into very advanced age. His book should be required reading for anyone who wants to be active and vital and stay that way for life. We share *The 100 Year Lifestyle* with our patients and community and it is making a huge impact."

Dr. Patricia McLean, a founder of League of Chiropractic Women and Dr. Michael S. McLean, FICA, President, International Chiropractors Association

"This Life Changing Bestseller is BACK and BETTER Than Ever"

Garrett B. Gunderson, *The New York Times® Bestselling Author*

Second Edition

The 100 Year Lifestyle

BREAKTHROUGH
SOLUTIONS
FOR REAL, LASTING, PERSONAL
AND CULTURAL CHANGE!

Live YOURS and Enjoy
Better Health, Healing, Energy,
Finances, Leadership, Faith,
Relationships and More -
Every Day Starting TODAY.

ERIC PLASKER, D.C., Internationally Acclaimed Health Expert
And Bestselling Author of *The 100 Year Lifestyle Workout*

Copyright © 2013, Dr. Eric Plasker
Published by LCFE, LLC
533 Johnson Ferry Road Suite C200
Marietta, GA 30068
www.100yearlifestyle.com
www.facebook.com/100yearlifestyle
www.youtube.com/user/100yearlifestyle
ISBN: 1475084609
ISBN: 9781475084603

FOREWORD

The 100 Year Lifestyle is an idea whose time has come. For you as an individual, this message can be life changing. For our culture, it represents an important new way of looking at health care and the way we view the world.

In this life changing book, Dr. Plasker has taken a 5,000 year old concept of Vitalism and made it SIMPLE for every individual who wants to optimize the expression of their inborn potential over the course of their entire lifetime.

Vitalism is the recognition that the universe and all living systems are conscience, self-developing, self-adapting and self-healing systems.

For 5000 years we have asked the question, "What is the nature of a human being?" Who are we? What are we made of? What is life? You might argue that you've never even entertained the idea much less landed on an answer. Yet, without intentional critical thinking, all of us by default without knowing it will automatically accept and live out an answer. That answer will determine the kind of health care system we create, the educational system we will send our children to, and the basic attitudes that underpin how we see others and the world we live in.

There have been essentially, two answers to the question. The first proposes that the universe is a big machine and we are likewise a machine made up exclusively of physical matter. In essence, that we can understand you, your needs and life itself by the chemistry and physics of the body.

This theory is called Atomism (made up of indivisible physical elements) or Mechanism (a machine). This is the default answer and our current health care system is built on this idea. So, we wait for the machine to break down, diagnose the bad part and then manipulate it back to medicine's version of "normal" with drugs and surgery. The major problem is that the machine is so complex that diagnosing is difficult at best, the organism can't be viewed as a set of independent parts, and consequently side effects occur throughout when we manipulate any one part.

The second theory is that we are vital beings. That life is more than chemistry and physics; that we are, in fact, self-developing (two half cells multiply in an intelligent way producing a whole human being), self-adapting (we are constantly adapting to an ever changing environment and health is the ability to successfully adapt), self-healing (the greatest scientist in the world can't create one living cell, but your body is constantly repairing and healing itself). This concept is called Vitalism and recognizes that life is intelligent and conscious; as such we are always developing higher levels of awareness, language, relationships, curiosity, etc.

If you accept the idea of Mechanism or Atomism then manipulating a person after they become sick with drugs and surgery is a logical conclusion.

Vitalism however proposes that we don't need to manipulate an intelligent system, but rather eliminate the interferences and the body will do what it was created to do...self-develop, adapt and heal. Vitalism would look to eliminate interferences like physical traumas, environmental toxins and emotional traumas, especially to the nervous system not only when a person has a health issue and wants a natural approach to recovery, but also as a means of prevention and optimizing their potential on every level.

So, you get to choose Mechanism or Vitalism. One has a great respect for the human body and its Innate Intelligence and believes that health comes from the inside out. The other believes that health is obtained through powders, pills and potions and that the doctor is giving health to you from the outside in. The consequences of your choice are profound....choose well.

The 100 Year Lifestyle tells us that the fastest growing segment of the population is those of us who will live to be 100. What will your last 20 years of life look like....a wheel chair, limited activity, mental lapses and few relationships or a vibrant active high quality of life? The problem is you can't sit by and hope for the best or think that it can be fixed when you get there.

At Life University we did a comprehensive study of people aged 15 to 30. Interestingly, these folks think they are going to be healthier than their parents and yet, their health behaviors are the same as their parents. We need to do something different and we need to do it now.

The 100 Year Lifestyle is that plan of action. For Doctors of Chiropractic and other true health care providers, it is a way to educate your patients and build your practice on the Vitalistic principles of chiropractic that stimulate lifelong patients bringing their kids in for care. It creates successful practices, but more importantly it creates meaningful practices that are significant and it has the potential to turn our health care paradigm around.

Life University is proud to be associated with this profound concept and movement.

Make your life extraordinary and you will enjoy a sensational century!

Guy Riekeman, DC, President, Life University

ACKNOWLEDGEMENTS

The 100 Year Lifestyle comes from both my inborn desire to help people, and a lifetime of experiences and relationships. I am thankful to all of the people who have contributed to my journey.

First and most importantly, I am thankful that God has blessed me with the talents and abilities to help so many people and make a difference.

Lisa, my wife of twenty-five years, thank you for believing in me, for standing by me as my partner in life, and for being an incredible mother to our children. I love you.

To my children, Jacob, Emily and Cory, I could never be more proud of you. Continue to search for your niche in the world and passionately apply yourself to the things that you love and the causes you believe in. Always remember to take care of yourselves and take care of each other. I love you all and I love being your dad.

My mom and dad are great parents and have given me so much over the years. Mom, thank you for passing your passion to me of wanting to help people reach their full potential. Dad, I wish you could read this book. You would be proud. Since you fell ill, my sense of urgency to complete this work has been accelerated. You have been such a strong, positive force in my life. I miss you very much.

My brothers, Drs. Jordan and Noel Plasker, are my best friends. You guys are an incredible source of strength for me. Seeing our kids love each other so much means the world to me.

To my mother and father in-law, Herb and Joanne Singer, thank you for embracing me into your family and loving my children.

I have been blessed with a huge family of cousins, many of whom are also some of my best friends in the world. There is no way to mention them all.

I have been blessed with so many great mentors and coaches over the years. From Ed Huber to Chuck Scarpula and Tony Amarillo, your leadership started me on the right track.

In my professional life, my mentors in chiropractic have been extraordinary. Dr. Ernie Landi, thank you for my first adjustment and for telling me the story. Drs. Alex, Doug and Jon Cox, thank you for your technical expertise and for teaching me to be an excellent doctor. Thanks to Dr. Guy Riekeman, President of Life University, for connecting me to the big idea and inspiring me to make a difference. It is an honor to work with the entire team at Life University to deliver this message to the masses. Dr. Joseph Flesia, you have impacted me more than anyone in my professional life. Your teachings and your memory inspire me every day. Just prior to the release of this book two of my most influential mentors passed away in Dr. Reggie Gold and Dr. Sid E. Williams. Both were in their mid-80s; however, both also lived 160 years in their 80 plus years of life.

My team at The Family Practice has given me incredible support including Teri Bynum-Kelly, Sergio Nascimento, Nyowo Scott and Kimberly Brenowitz.

Thanks also to all of our 100 Year Lifestyle Licensed Affiliate Chiropractors who are committed to delivering The 100 Year Lifestyle as a health care model to the people of their community. Special thanks to the following doctors who have contributed their voice and thoughts to this Second Edition including: Dr. Jay Handt, Dr. Josh Handt and Dr. Morgan Handt, Dr. Dan Mosier, Dr. Jack Bourla,

Dr. John Bueler, Dr. Dennis Buckley, Dr. Rebecca Wilson, Drs. Brent and Devin Waterman, Drs. Jennifer and Stephanie Rozenhart, Dr. Andrew Burns, Dr. Norm Colby and Dr. Cathy Wendland-Colby, Drs. Glenn and Aryn Gabai, Dr. Kevin Joe, Dr. Lyle Koca, Dr. Glenn Lang, Dr. Jamie Lucia, Drs. Pat and Mike McLean, Dr. David Moore, Dr. Brandon Roberts, Dr. Vincent Punturere, Dr. Aixa Goodrich, Dr. Jim Dubel, Dr. Sam Selimo, Dr. Tony DeMarco, Dr. Bill Henry, Dr. Robert Tarantino. In addition I continue to have gratitude towards the doctors who contributed their heart to The 100 Year Lifestyle First Edition including Dr. Cheryl Langley, Dr. Carmelo Caratozzolo, Dr. Russ Pavkov, Dr. Gary Brodeur, Dr. Tina Theriot, Dr. Bart Rzepa, Dr. Craig Pruitt, Dr. Miguel Cruz, Dr. Scott Stachelek, and Dr. Terry Harmon, lets continue to grow by helping as many people as possible to reach their full health potential.

Thank you to all of my thousands of patients over the years who taught me about health and healing, human potential, hope and possibility. Your belief in me nurtured the seeds of this book and made me realize the importance of taking a stand for people.

Thank you to my good friends and mentors over the years who have touched my life including Dr. Brian Kelly, Dr. Brian McCauley, Dr. Edwin Cordero, Dr. Fabrizio Mancini, Mark Victor Hansen, Jack Canfield, Barbara De Angelis, Dan Sullivan, Dr. Bob Hoffman, Dr. Gerald Clum, Dr. Ari Diskin, Stedman Graham to name a few.

The list can go on and on and I am grateful to all of the people in my life who are living The 100 Year Lifestyle and committed to expressing their Innate potential. The vision continues to expand because of you. Together we are making the world a healthier place for all of us.

Now let's take it up another notch on our way to a sensational century.

TABLE OF CONTENTS

THE 100 YEAR LIFESTYLE ASSESSMENT:
TAKE THE LIFESTYLE LEAP!

Are you living The 100 Year Lifestyle or The 50 – 60 Year Lifestyle? Find out by honestly answering the following questions about your current life. Your state of mind may be good, or bad, today. Regardless of how you feel in the moment, please give these simple questions a little bit more thoughtfulness to get your real score!

1 means Never and 5 means Always.

I am excited about the possibility of living to 100

1	2	3	4	5

I have many goals that I would like to achieve over my extended life

1	2	3	4	5

I am willing to make changes to improve my quality of life as I age

1	2	3	4	5

I have youthful energy in spite of my age

1	2	3	4	5

I enjoy a full night of restful sleep and feel energized each morning

1	2	3	4	5

I can consciously shift my energy whenever I want

1	2	3	4	5

I am aware of the diseases in my family history

1	2	3	4	5

I live a lifestyle that counteracts the diseases in my family history

1	2	3	4	5

I am motivated by quality of life health goals rather than crisis

1	2	3	4	5

I feel good about my current health condition and do not rely on prescription or non-prescription drugs

1	2	3	4	5

I exercise 4 to 5 times a week and am getting the results I want from my fitness routine

1	2	3	4	5

I eat healthy and supplement my diet

| 1 | 2 | 3 | 4 | 5 |

I visit health care providers proactively to stay healthy and avoid unnecessary health problems

| 1 | 2 | 3 | 4 | 5 |

I live in a peaceful, stress-free home environment

| 1 | 2 | 3 | 4 | 5 |

I work in an environment that nurtures my talents and where I feel appreciated

| 1 | 2 | 3 | 4 | 5 |

My home and work environment reflect my inner feelings and voice

| 1 | 2 | 3 | 4 | 5 |

I support myself through choices that I know are good for me

| 1 | 2 | 3 | 4 | 5 |

I actively seek out opportunities and enjoy learning new things

| 1 | 2 | 3 | 4 | 5 |

I am surrounded by supportive relationships at home and at work

| 1 | 2 | 3 | 4 | 5 |

I have achieved the balance I am looking for

| 1 | 2 | 3 | 4 | 5 |

I am able to separate work time from Play Time

| 1 | 2 | 3 | 4 | 5 |

I have a clear picture of how I want to use my time during my extended life

| 1 | 2 | 3 | 4 | 5 |

My current financial path can sustain me until I reach 100

| 1 | 2 | 3 | 4 | 5 |

I am passionate about work and the way I earn money

| 1 | 2 | 3 | 4 | 5 |

I am living within my means and investing in myself and my future

| 1 | 2 | 3 | 4 | 5 |

I feel like my life has purpose and I am making a difference

| 1 | 2 | 3 | 4 | 5 |

I am actively involved in my community

| 1 | 2 | 3 | 4 | 5 |

I have a mentor and I use my leadership skills to mentor others

| 1 | 2 | 3 | 4 | 5 |

Add all the circled numbers. This is your total score: _____

WHAT YOUR SCORE MEANS

If your score was 0 to 35: Slam On The Brakes and Change Your Life. You are either in denial, at the end of your ropes, or just don't care. At the rate you are going both your mind and your body are headed for trouble. You are taking years off your life and will be a financial burden to your children or society. It's not too late to turn things around. Keep reading and embrace the Three Life Changing Principles of The 100 Year Lifestyle to make the remaining years of your life the best. Take the Lifestyle Leap and pay close attention to the Three Life Changing Principles in Chapter 2!

If your score was 36 to 70: Stop Killing Yourself Slowly. At the rate you are going you are headed for a deteriorating and depressing extended life. You have no vision, poor habits, and lack a sense of purpose. You are using crisis as the motivation to take action on the habits that you know are good for you, rather than embracing the quality of life you deserve. Stop compromising yourself. You can simply, steadily, and easily make 100 Year Lifestyle changes to enjoy your longevity with the health, passion, and meaning to make it all worthwhile. Take the Lifestyle Leap and enjoy the youthful energy and enthusiasm that you will learn about in Chapters 3 and 4!

If your score was 71 to 105: Get Ready to Go from Good to Great. You are probably on a roller coaster filled with ups and downs. You are enjoying your life, but you are out of balance with swings that go too far to the extreme. Some things are working well for you, while other areas of your life are out of control. Address the areas of The 100 Year Lifestyle that will impact your life the most and you will find that your life gets easier, your results go up, and you start having a lot more fun. You will add better health, financial security, peace of mind, and purpose to an already solid foundation. Take the Lifestyle Leap and discover how to attract new friends, find new passions, and achieve the balance you are looking for by embracing the ideas in Chapters 14, 15, 16 and 17!

If your score was 106-140: Enjoy a Sensational Century. You are on your way. You are living your dreams while you plan for the future, both at the same time. You enjoy your work and feel like you can do it forever. The good news is that by following this plan, it won't be something you have to do, but something you can choose to do if you want to. You are in good health, you have goals to achieve, and a world of opportunity lies ahead of you. Embracing The 100 Year Lifestyle will ensure that you enjoy your legacy while you are alive, enjoy youthful energy and passion, and make the most of this precious gift called your life. Take the Lifestyle Leap by refining your life vision, having more fun than ever, and making your life matter by adopting the concepts in Chapters 17, 19 and 20!

INTRODUCTION

Over the past 6 years, we've witnessed terroristic attacks, wars, Hurricane Sandy, another recession, a new president who was then re-elected, and for many, the worst economy we've seen in our lifetime and yet, we are still here. Many of us have experienced the loss of loved ones, including me with my father's passing. Some of us have gone through major life changes like divorce, graduating with a new degree, getting married, the loss of a job or becoming the main caregiver for an aging parent or grandparent and yet, we are still here.

While those changes were occurring, the United State rankings declined in key areas of Life Expectancy and Infant Mortality and yet, you and I are still here.

Are you living your best life? Are you making things happen and making the changes you know you need to make or are you procrastinating and avoiding the obvious? What are you waiting for?

On a personal note, I've seen my children grow into responsible adults and I feel a greater sense of wisdom, a knowing, that the principles of The 100 Year Lifestyle are enduring. They will continue to lead a revolution of lasting personal and cultural change!

Since the release of The 100 Year Lifestyle, the book and its principles enjoyed a rapid ascent up the Bestseller list. It has been translated into several languages and is being read worldwide. The 100 Year Lifestyle Workout book became the #1 fitness book upon its release and has become a great reference tool, and a catalyst, for people to get in the best shape of their lives. The 100 Year Lifestyle

YouTube channel and The 100 Year Lifestyle fan page on Facebook are engaging people and keeping this life changing conversation ongoing.

The 100 Year Lifestyle health care philosophy and chiropractic practice model is helping individuals around the world find quality health care in a model they can trust. I continue to be inspired by the stories of people who are changing their lives. From individuals losing over 300 pounds to people starting a new business and growing their practices, the 100 Year Lifestyle model remains a catalyst and an anchor for individuals who want to express their full potential for a lifetime. It defines a new model for living in a world of extended life spans.

If you knew you'd live to 100, how would you change your life? One of the world's most famous centenarians, George Burns, summed it up well when he joked that had he known he was going to live to be 100, he would have taken better care of himself. Never has a punch line more profoundly put the aging process in the proper perspective! Let this irony open the doorway to smart choices that can support you in every way as your genealogy edges you toward the increasing probability that you will live to 100 or longer!

As a dedicated chiropractor, corporate and municipal health care consultant, health and wellness expert, columnist, and lecturer for a quarter century, I have been a catalyst in helping people of all ages maximize the quality and quantity of their lives. They've done it by practicing the Life Changing Principles I've developed over the past two decades of researching and probing the depths of human potential. Coined a "Change Master" by my colleagues and patients, it's my mission to give you life-enhancing information that generates real transformation in your level of health, prosperity, and happiness.

The truth is staggering. Anyone who is 40 years of age today could live to be 100 years old and their grandchildren could live even longer than that. While this information is exciting to me and to many of my clients, I am taken aback by the large number of people who express a reluctance to ride this road for fear they'll out-live their assets, experience declining health, or be a burden to their family. Unwilling to compromise on my own quality of life as I age, I dedicated my career to teaching audiences around the world how to change their lives and embrace this new lease on longevity and minimize any of its ill effects.

The truth is your body has the hardware to live healthy to 80, 90, 100 years and beyond. It was imbedded in your Innate Intelligence from the moment of your conception. Understanding and accept-ing this Innate opportunity will help you express your unlimited life potential. The 100 Year Lifestyle strategies you uncover in this book will not only help you embrace an extended life span, but teach you how to live life to the fullest every day and live your best possible legacy while you are alive, rather than just leave it after you are gone.

How will you accept this gift of extra time? Will it be with grati-tude or reluctance and more importantly, how will this gift inspire you to change your career, family relationships, and life priorities?

How will it impact the way you raise your children, as today's generation of kids may be the first in recent history to see their life expectancy go down, not because of their genes, but because of their lifestyle choices? Together, we will uncover the anatomy of your extended life span as well as the health, energy, and riches that can be yours as a result of this gift.

If you're going to live to 80, 90, or 100 years and beyond anyway, why not make it a sensational century? Elevate your consciousness and choose to change the way you view, plan, manage, and live your life. Put these inspiring and life-changing principles into place and optimize your health, wealth, and professional and personal relationships. Create a signature life plan that will prepare you physically, financially, and emotionally to live a joyous life no matter what your age every step of the way. The 100 Year Lifestyle will give you the mindset, knowledge and tools for living an incredible life every day of your life for 80, 90, 100 years and beyond.

Enjoy the journey!

Dr. Eric Plasker

Founder of The Family Practice, Inc., and LCfE, LLC

www.100yearlifestyle.com

www.facebook.com/100yearlifestyle

www.youtube.com/user/100yearlifestyle

PART 1

Welcome to The 100 Year Lifestyle

*If I knew I was going
to live this long,
I would have…*

CHAPTER 1

TELL ME SOMETHING I DON'T KNOW

Welcome to The 100 Year Lifestyle. I'll bet this isn't the first book you've purchased hoping to improve the quality of your life. In fact, our world is filled with so much information on the Internet and in the book stores that you may even think you already know all there is to know about building a life of lasting health, wealth, and meaningful relationships. "Tell me something I don't know," you say.

But, there's a reason why you bought this book. There's a reason why you, like many of our readers, may be reading this for the second, third or fourth time. Could it be that your life is at a crossroads? Did you just have a milestone birthday or anniversary? Have you had to place a beloved parent or grandparent in a nursing home? Did you recently attend a funeral? Maybe you're feeling younger than ever regardless of your age and you want to optimize the opportunities that lie ahead of you. Or maybe your feeling older than you should and you're ready to rediscover your youthful energy and passion for life. Maybe you recently had children and are realizing that your choices are not just about you anymore and you need to adjust your lifestyle and change your priorities. Is it possible that up until now, the messages you've received haven't been meaningful enough to get you to take action? Has changing just seemed like more trouble than it's worth?

Now, let me tell you something you may not know. Change is easy; it's thinking about change that is hard. When you finally have the realization that your parents' and grandparents' generation is living nearly twice as long as scientists thought they would, and you probably will too, what will you do about it? Will this be the catalyst for you to make the changes you know you need to make to ensure the quality of life you want and deserve? Will you start taking better care of yourself physically, mentally, socially, and financially? Are you ready to get excited about the rest of your life?

In this book, you are going to find a blueprint for living your best life every day, starting with today, to 80, 90, 100 years—and beyond with health and vitality. The focus is on helping you to identify and optimize your own unique, Innate Intelligence. It's a fascinating journey and I'm honored to accompany you through it.

Along the way, you will embrace some exciting new concepts and realities about human potential, aging and longevity that are life changing. For example, like it or not, the fact is that our grandparents' generation is living nearly twice as long as scientists thought they would. They were unprepared for this good fortune and many have paid the price for it. They didn't think that they would need their health, finances, or relationships to sustain them for so long and as a result, they haven't. *For this reason, very few of us regard old age as something positive.*

You are about to begin seeing things a different way. You'll even meet 90-year-olds and centenarians, who are already living The 100 Year Lifestyle today, such as Henry Rohlfs of Short Hills, New Jersey, who celebrated his ninetieth birthday by taking a ride in a hot air balloon over Luxor, Egypt. I wonder what kind of adventures you will choose to make the most of all the decades that you have left.

You will discover in this book that managing your health is a lot like managing your money. Good intentions are not enough—you must back them up with actions. This is so important because if the experts are right and the current aging trends continue, you'll probably end up living much longer than you ever imagined but will they be quality years? That may depend on your choices today!

There is tremendous opportunity in The 100 Year Lifestyle which will be revealed to you. By planning for your own longevity, you are opening the door to the opportunity of not only "first" and "second" acts, but "third" and "fourth" acts as well. You are opening the door to an abundance of new beginnings, knowing that there is time to accomplish every goal you've ever dreamed of. You'll substitute refinement for retirement as you maintain a sense of productivity, purpose, and passion for life—throughout your entire lifetime.

THE 100 YEAR LIFESTYLE DEFINED:

What it is...

- Living a healthy, passionate, prosperous life, every day of your life, for 100 years and beyond
- Great relationships with multiple generations and multiple circles of people
- Lifelong learning, activity, and adventure
- Keeping your spine and nervous system functioning without interference so you can adapt to your environment and function at your full potential
- Financial freedom, abundance, and independence
- The perfect balance of exploration, Play Time, and fun combined with meaningful work
- Optimizing your Innate capabilities and making the most of your time, energy, and talents

- Keeping your original body parts functioning at full capacity and keeping your mind sharp
- Accepting challenges, embracing change, and adapting to the unexpected
- Balancing the need for immediate gratification and a secure future
- Knowing and trusting yourself
- Yours to customize

What it is not...

- Rotting away as a human preservative in a nursing home
- Abusing your body, masking symptoms with drugs, and then continuing to abuse yourself until one organ after the other has to be removed or replaced
- All work and no play
- Abusive relationships or isolation
- Financial survival for 35 years and then barely squeaking by on Social Security and Medicare
- Insignificant retirement where you become a meaningless number in a long line of an outdated system
- Wearing out your body in the first 50 years and then suffering the consequences during the second 50 years
- Accumulating wealth in the first 50 years and destroying relationships along the way, leaving you nobody to share it with Creating wealth at the price of your health
- Denying yourself the good things in life

Understand that life expectancy and life span are two different things. Prior to the twentieth century, life expectancy was about half of what it is today, but the life span was not that different. Many people have been documented as living beyond 90 as far back as the sixteenth century.

What is happening today is that more and more people are experiencing longevity in their natural life spans. This is great news, but only when you are able to enjoy a good quality of life—throughout your life. And what you will see in this book is that actions leading to a healthy, abundant 100 Year Lifestyle will also optimize the quality of your life today.

It's a fact that centenarians—people who are living to 100 or more—are one of the fastest-growing age groups in the United States and many other industrialized nations around the world. When the first edition of The 100 Year Lifestyle was written, there were an estimated 50,000 centenarians in the United States. There are now over 70,000 centenarians living in this country. The number is climbing! If you are a baby boomer, you'll join the nearly 400 million people around the world who will be 80 years of age or older by 2050 and the estimated 2 million centenarians in the United States alone. Are you ready for this incredible opportunity? Will you enjoy the quality of life that you deserve along the way?

I've spent the last quarter of a century asking thousands of patients, doctors and seminar attendees one powerful question, "If you knew you'd live to 100, how would you change your life?" To my surprise, many of them express no desire to live that long. They worry that they will run out of money. They worry they will end up isolated and alone. They don't want to be a cripple or a burden to their family and friends.

So, how do you plan to approach this potential milestone? Will you keep overworking and under-exercising? Will you eat more than you should and be less fulfilled than you could be? Or will you make the most of your journey along the way?

Will knowing that you have the ability to live a century or more lend urgency to your desire to change the way you approach your own life? A lot of it depends on how you respond to what you think you already know.

Throughout this book, I will give you opportunities to take action on our discussions through Live Long and Strong exercises. Take the action steps and get involved in the process to customize your own 100 Year Lifestyle. No one else can live it for you.

LIVE LONG AND STRONG

If you knew you were going to live to 100, how would you change your life?

List the immediate changes that you know deep down in your heart that you need to make:
1._____
2._____
3._____
4._____
5._____

What are the long-term and lasting changes you would make?
1._____
2._____
3._____
4._____
5._____

CRISIS MOTIVATION VERSUS QUALITY-OF-LIFE MOTIVATION

We live in a society where crisis motivates us to change. It takes a heart attack to get many people to stop smoking or to eat healthy. When we can't fit into our clothes anymore, we decide to cut calories or to start exercising. It's a paradoxical health approach where illness inspires us to be well. It's one that may leave you punching the nurse call button instead of enjoying the active, healthy lifestyle you deserve.

About twenty years ago, a 98-year-old man walked into my chiropractic office in Atlanta. His name was Max and he was beautiful old man who was in severe, miserable pain. His level of suffering was extreme and he had been suffering on some level since the age of 50. He shuffled in with a bent back and arthritic fingers. It hurt just to look at him. Unable to stand upright, Max told me he couldn't bear the pain much longer and he was ready to do whatever it took to improve his quality of life. I could not believe he waited so long to see a chiropractor.

After nearly a year of gentle adjustments, Max's discomfort had mostly subsided. His flexibility and mobility improved, and he was extremely grateful for his new lease on life. His Crisis Care was complete, and Max stopped coming in. For months, my staff made attempts to re-engage him in the Critical Transition phase of his care, but Max was nowhere to be found. We couldn't contact him by phone, and there were no family members that we could reach. The letters we mailed went unanswered. Eventually, we gave up. Max was now 99 years old and we assumed he had passed.

A year later, I was surprised to find Max, who was now over 100 years old, standing in my doorway. As I got closer to him, I could see that he was weak and tired. He looked like a man who was ready to pass. He looked up at me and said, "Thank you Dr. Plasker, thank you", and then collapsed on the counter in my reception room and died. Sadness and shock spread through my office as the ambulance drove him away. There was nobody to call and no family to console. I understood then why Max had come to my office. He had come there because he had no other place to go.

Max had lived to the 100 year mark with no money, no physical strength, no energy, and no loving connections to sustain him. On the surface, it seemed like there was nothing left of Max. But the truth is he left something huge behind for me.

It was a question mark so large that I could not ignore it. The question was, "If Max had known he was going to live to 100, how would he have changed his life when he was 20, 30, 40, 50, or 60 years old so that he didn't get there crippled, broke and alone?" Would he have made his health, wealth, and relationships a priority at a much younger age?

What could he have accomplished if he nurtured his passion, potential and relationships along the way?

You and I both know there is a better way. Living to 100 doesn't have to mean outliving your resources, relationships, or joy. In fact, you'll find many older Americans working out at the gym, dancing at parties, and traveling the globe. Just look at Jack LaLanne, the Godfather of Fitness who helped people to change and improve their lifestyle. He continued to inspire up until his passing at age 96. What an honor it was to share speaking and media platforms with him on many occasions. He inspired me so much.

Fauja Singh, a British 101 year old, marathon runner, and torch bearer during the 2012 Olympics, began running at age 89 to remain occupied and active after his wife and son had passed away. Mr. Singh said, "The secret to a long and healthy life is to be stress-free. Be grateful for everything you have, stay away from people who are negative, stay smiling and keep running."

These people let their love for life—and desire to be healthy—motivate their choices. They have not let crisis be their catalyst for living their ideal 100 Year Lifestyle.

The truth is nobody wants to be forced into anything—especially change. We resent it when we don't choose our path freely.

I'll bet at some time or another, you've gone to your closet to get dressed and found a pair of pants that no longer fits. This forces you to do one of two things—both of which you are likely to resent. One, you could go out and buy new clothes. Or two, you could go on a diet to lose the extra weight. As a result of being forced into either decision, you likely became resentful. You resent the change that is required to resolve the problem.

My father is an example of someone who was forced to change. He changed the way he ate, exercised, and took care of his body after he had a heart attack. While he was thankful to get a second chance, he did not take up running because it was a pleasurable, proactive way to improve his health. He ran to save his life.

Wouldn't it be better if you chose change not because you had to, but because you care about you? Allowing quality of life—and not crisis—to motivate you makes changing easier, more exciting, and more fun while helping you to avoid unnecessary detours along the way.

TAKE ACTION ON YOUR RESOLUTIONS

How many times have you made a New Year's resolution to lose weight, get in shape, start investing, take a vacation, or spend more time with your loved ones? How long were you able to keep your commitments? Right now, I want you to forget about these previous attempts and start fresh. It doesn't matter whether you've started a dozen diets and stopped, tried to resign from a dead-end job and backed down, or made it only two minutes when you were trying to meditate. This book is going to show you how to put life changing principles to work for you without all the hesitation or heartbreak any past attempts may have had. I am not going to let you do a last-minute scramble to regain what you could have kept all along.

If you really believe you cannot change the quality of your life today or in the future, then go ahead and close this book. You can just keep doing the same things you always do and getting the same things you always get, or you can allow me to escort you into the best years of your life.

TAKING ADVANTAGE OF THE ODDS

Perhaps you are not ready to believe in the fact that you're likely to see your hundredth birthday. You may not even want to live to 100. You may find the thought of it depressing. However, your resistance won't change the fact that your odds of getting there are greater than ever. Very few, if any, of our current centenarians wanted to get their either, but they got their anyway.

It's not enough for me—or the news media—to throw information at you. This will not motivate you to change. You have to want what is rightfully yours. You have to want to be well. You've got to want to optimize your health and express your Innate potential. It's not enough to simply avoid sickness. You have to want to live the quality life that deep down you know you deserve. Changing your mind about how long you can—and probably will—live opens up a whole world of opportunity. This new paradigm brings better health, fuller coffers, and richer relationships as a result of your acceptance of this wondrous gift. Align yourself with this true view of your Innate potential and it will be hard for anyone or anything to pull you off course.

The U.S. Census Bureau reported 13 percent of Americans were over 65 in 2011 and the projected world population change between 2005-2040 for people 100 or older will be 746 percent. More than half of all the babies born since 2000 can expect to live to 100, according to The Lancet, BMJ. The MacArthur Foundation has determined that only 30 percent of aging is based on genetics while 70 percent is attributed to lifestyle choices.

These findings mean living to 100 is not just for a select few, but for you and me as well. It means that evolution and advances in self-care and health care are giving you a wakeup call to your God-given birthright. It is a gift of extra time to accomplish all your goals, nurture your relationships, master your areas of interest, and contribute more to the world. Knowing that you really do have all the time you need to reach your destination could even stop your "urgency addiction" of rushing from one point to the next. It's a gift that can give you the strength and patience to take on even the most exciting and challenging opportunities in your life. In fact, if you make your lifestyle changes now, you will be able to enjoy the results of those changes for decades.

How well would you say your biological clock has been keeping time? Are you feeling or looking older than you'd like? Are there aspects of yourself you'd like to change? No matter where you are in your 100 year journey so far, it is not time to slow down or "settle" for any one thing or place in life. But, it is time to get your mind onboard with what you now know your biology can do and embrace the reality of your longevity with passion.

ADVANCE NOTICE ON AGING

When was the last time you looked through your family photo albums? Take them out and look at your mother and father when they were your age. Look at their parents when they were younger, too. Now think about how they aged. Look at their skin and their posture. How severely did their activity decline as they aged? Did they become crippled by preventable health problems such as arthritis, osteoporosis, or heart disease?

The number of people who are affected by these and many other preventable health conditions is staggering. Twenty-seven million people are affected by osteoarthritis in the United States. Approximately 35 percent of adults older than 65 are obese and another 33 percent are overweight, putting them at substantially increased risk for diabetes, hypertension, heart disease, and other illnesses. Many health conditions that we take for granted in this country are not a normal part of aging elsewhere. They are largely brought on by our lifestyle—by our choices.

Visit www.youtube.com/user/100yearlifestyle and watch "You Inherited a Lifestyle."

So, now it's time to take a good look at you. Scan your own reflection in the mirror. How are your skin, bones, and waistline? In what kind of shape are your heart, lungs, liver, and kidneys? How is your posture, straight and strong, or are you beginning to show signs of imbalance, swayback or hunching over? Is your spine aligned and is your nerve system functioning properly? If you continue on your current path, will you like the way you age? Can you imagine your photograph in twenty, thirty, or forty years? Embracing The 100 Year Lifestyle will ensure that you blossom today, now and over the remaining decades that lie ahead of you.

What did your parents and grandparents know about their own aging potential? When today's centenarians were born, science only gave them a life expectancy of 50 years. They were blindsided by their longevity. During their lifetimes, their life expectancies doubled without warning. They had no vision and no strategy for their extended lives. What a surprise it must be for them to find themselves still living. None of them ever thought they could live to 100, but their bodies did it regardless of what they believed. No wonder many of them sit around as grumpy old people. How do you get when you are a week or a month late on a project? Doesn't this cause you to be angry or frustrated? Can you imagine if you were 30, 40, or 50 years late for your funeral?

This generation that Tom Brokaw calls "the Greatest Generation" has lived through World War I and World War II, developed the automobile and airplane, sent humans to the moon, and managed to outlive their predicted life span by five decades! They have watched in disbelief as technology moved center stage—with the advent of the radio, then television, computers, and the Internet. Just as technology has advanced, so has the length of their lives. They are reaching record longevity in spite of what they thought they knew to be true.

Your grandparents and parents weren't taught that their bodies were designed to live 100 years or more. They weren't taught how to prepare for their longevity. Many of them didn't cultivate physical, mental or financial stability to ensure a hundred or more quality years. This "Greatest Generation" is now giving you your greatest gift. They are giving you a preview of what awaits you as a result of your ability to live longer and wiser than any generation before you.

Centenarian Secret
Aging poorly is not inevitable. You do have a choice. Based on your parents' and grandparents' experiences, you'll see where you're headed unless you choose a different path.

THE ACCIDENTAL CENTENARIANS

The majority of today's centenarians never thought about how they would approach their later years because they never expected to have them. They got there by accident. This "Greatest Generation" is now paying the greatest price for not knowing. In fact, many of them are paying over $10,000 a month to live in nursing homes. They have gone from Greatest Generation to Nursing Home Generation and assisted living centers are popping up everywhere to house this blindsided bunch.

These seniors were simply not prepared for such an extended stay here on earth. They believed that if they worked for 35 or 40 years, they could live off of their Social Security benefits, pensions or retirement funds for their remaining 10 to 20 years maximum, and then they would die. The truth is those resources now need to last twice as long. Our government is grappling with the consequences of this quandary as they are now scrambling to try and save Social Security and Medicare.

We are the first generation in history that is getting this advance notice. This is your advance notice! What will you do with this information?

Visit www.youtube.com/user/100yearlifestyle and watch "The First Generation Ever."

Living The 100 Year Lifestyle
Madame Jeanne Calment lived a 100 Year Lifestyle. She reportedly took up fencing at 85, was still riding her bike at 100, and released a rap CD at 121 years of age. She was still learning, growing, and staying physically active as she reached and surpassed the 100 Year mark.

In search of purpose, passion, and a little extra cash, many seniors are going back to work in the latter part of their lives. They find the field of opportunity really opens up during their "Second Act" since money is oftentimes no longer their primary motivation.

Older Americans are also heading back to school in droves. Nearly 435,000 Americans 50-plus years of age and older are now part-time college students. Another 120,000 are working toward graduate degrees and 85,000 are full-time college students. According to a recent survey by U.S. News and World Report, the number of college students ages 40 to 64 has increased nearly 20% to almost two million in the last decade. Compare this active, happy, lifestyle to the 86-year-old mother of a patient of mine. She fell and broke her hip last year. Since then, her health has been declining quickly. Every time the daughter's phone rings, she panics. She knows it will be another issue with her mom. She prays her mother has not broken another hip or lost another ten pounds. She prays she will not grow old the same way her mother has.

This book is about making choices that will support the quality of your longevity—today and tomorrow. Honor the life you have been given by making the most of the time you have. The fact is that if you are living life to the fullest, maxing out your potential, and enjoying your most important relationships, your life is going to feel pretty short. Even if it lasts beyond 100, it will feel like it is flying by.

Keep your vision in sync with your biology. Calibrate your vision with your extended life span to ensure that the quality matches the quantity of your years. The power of this paradigm shift will give you the ability to write the remaining chapters of your life—with the best ones still to come.

Innate Life Expectancy
Calculate Your M-PYR

Here's how to calculate your Minimum Potential Years Remaining, your M-PYR (pronounced "empire"):

1. What was/is the age of your oldest grandparent ever?   _____
2. What is your current age?   _____
3. Your M-PYR is #1 minus #2   _____

Now, do the calculation again using your spouse's or your child's current age instead of yours. What is their M-PYR? _____

Your M-PYR is not your MAX-PYR, or maximum potential years remaining. Who knows what your number could be? If you eat healthy, exercise, take care of your structure, spine and nervous system, nurtured good relationships and felt a sense of purpose, what would be the limits of your longevity?

Watch "Your Minimum Potential Years Remaining" and "Your Family's M-PYR" at www.youtube.com/user/100yearlifestyle. If you would like to share this with your friends and family, invite them to visit www.100yearlifestyle.com and select the M-PYR Calculator.

Remember the findings from the British Medical Journal, the *Lancet*, that 50 percent of the babies born since the year 2000 are expected to live over the age of 100? Additional research is concerned that our current generation of children may be the first generation in recent history to see their life expectancy go down.

How can this be? Doesn't it seem like a contradiction to see so many children living longer than ever while, as a society, their overall life expectancy goes down? The answer is sad yet simple in that the other 50 percent of children are expected to die younger and sicker than ever, not because of their genetics, but because of their unhealthy lifestyle choices.

Adjust your lifestyle today. If you are a parent, adjust your children's lifestyle. They need your healthy leadership. Lead them. Your parenting choices will impact your children's lives for decades, and maybe even after you are gone. Living The 100 Year Lifestyle will ensure that your children get on track for living their best life every day.

A NEW WAY OF AGING

It's no wonder that so many people have anxiety about aging. *The Merriam-Webster Dictionary* defines it as "a declining phase of life." However, today's pre-centenarians and post-centenarians are reinventing our notion of aging. Like former U.S. President George H. Bush who celebrated his 70th birthday by going skydiving, many seniors are pushing the limits of their Innate potential and loving every minute of it, realizing that they have plenty of time left to live their life!

Today's centenarians are teaching us that growing older is not a one-way ticket to deterioration and inactivity. They are showing us a new way of aging that is full of excitement and opportunity if you combine the right attitude with the right actions.

How do you feel about your life experience so far? Are you excited about your present and future? Would a change of personal habits, residence, relationships, career, health, or finances improve your level of happiness and prosperity? Will the choices you make today enable you to look back with no regrets when you are 80, 90 or 100?

I know you know the things you need to change. "Yes," you say, "I know it is easier to be fit than fat. I know it is easier to be solvent than bankrupt. I know it is better to be in love than alone." But, what are you doing with what you know? Don't you think it's time to stop just thinking about it and to start acting on change? You do have time to turn things around and take things to the next level. Let's get started.

CHAPTER 2

THE THREE LIFE-CHANGING PRINCIPLES OF THE 100 YEAR LIFESTYLE

Are you still with me? Great. You are on your way to living your best life, every day of your life, for 80, 90, 100 years and beyond.

We'll begin by embracing the changes you know you need to make. In the chapters ahead, you'll discover how to access the energy to fuel your longevity while ending all the old habits, patterns, and behaviors that are keeping you from living your best life every day. You will then become healthier than you've ever been before and put a team in place to sustain that health for a lifetime. Next, you'll create an ideal environment and support system for your extended life and set yourself up to enjoy the journey more than ever. You'll learn how to achieve balance, finance your 100 Year Lifestyle and enjoy your best life every step of the way.

At the core of customizing your 100 Year Lifestyle are these three Life Changing Principles that you will use throughout this journey:

The Three Life Changing Principles of The 100 Year Lifestyle
Life Changing Principle #1: Change is easy. Thinking about change is hard.
Life Changing Principle #2: Change happens one choice at a time. Think progress, not perfection.
Life Changing Principle #3: Approach change with your ideal 100 Year Lifestyle in mind.

These principles will make change exciting and achievable. They will empower you to age constructively instead of destructively. They will help you make your life so much more than before because the odds are you are going to have nearly a century or more to mold your life into everything you've always wanted it to be.

LIFE CHANGING PRINCIPLE #1:
CHANGE IS EASY—THINKING ABOUT CHANGE IS HARD

You've probably already experienced this: Resisting change is much harder than embracing it.

If you've ever played with magnets, you can understand the power behind Life Changing Principle #1. When you hold two magnets near each other with the like poles pointed toward each other, they repel one another no matter how hard you try to make the two ends meet. However, once you flip their orientation so the opposite charges are facing each other, they effortlessly attract and stick together. Then, instead of requiring energy to hold them together, it takes enormous energy to pull the magnets apart.

The magnet experiment is a metaphor for how we experience change once we commit to it. I see this play out in my patients and clients who continue with bad habits that force them to expend excess energy just to keep their lives together—knowing that it would be less effort if they just went ahead and chose a healthier path. I love watching the pieces of their lives fall effortlessly into place once they commit to change. It is a spiritual and physical demonstration of Life Changing Principle #1 and how change is easy. It's the thinking about it that is hard.

It used to be thought that if you had a family history of heart disease or cancer then it was your destiny to get these conditions too because they were "in your genes." Through the science of Epi-genetics we are learning that nothing can be further from the truth. Epi-genetics, which means 'around the gene', has shown that your lifestyle choices, both positive and negative, can influence the expression of your genes.

A recent report in the journal *Proceeding of the National Academy of Sciences USA* found the activity of more than 500 genes in the normal tissue of thirty men with low-risk prostate cancer changed after the patients began eating diets higher in fruits, vegetables and whole grains and lower in red meats and fats while also implementing an exercise and stress reducing regimen.

After three months the men had changes in the activity of about 500 genes including 48 disease preventing genes that were turned on and 453 disease promoting genes that were turned off.

I Changed My Course of History – Amber Eckel, DC

In 2009, I felt a lump in my thyroid gland during our physical exam skills class. I knew something was wrong. I've always been one to trust my Innate, so I sought out medical attention from my doctor back in Canada that summer. I didn't have any family history of thyroid disease, nor was I experiencing symptoms so my doctor thought it was unlikely that anything would actually be wrong. I asked to get an ultrasound anyway. After the first ultrasound, my doctor reported a 1 cm nodule on the left lobe of my thyroid. She also stated that thyroid nodules are fairly common, and 95 percent are non-cancerous. She then recommended that I get another ultrasound ~ 6 months later to ensure that the nodule wasn't growing. Unfortunately, after the second ultrasound, the nodule measured 1.4 cm, and thus she recommended a biopsy a few days later.

One month later, I was told I had thyroid cancer. This shocked me. I loved life and lived it to the fullest, but I had just been diagnosed with cancer. Later in 2010, I was told that my surgeon would need to remove the left lobe of my thyroid. Although the biopsy was positive, my surgeon insisted to only take out the affected side as he didn't fully believe that I had papillary carcinoma because I was young, healthy, symptom-less, and had not family history of any thyroid conditions. After the surgery, and confirmation that it was in fact papillary carcinoma, he instructed me that he would then have to do a 2nd surgery to remove the right lobe of my thyroid, as there is a "high" chance of reoccurrence. I was devastated that I had to go through this traumatic surgery again, and that I would have to be put on a thyroid medication for the rest of my life! Luckily, between the 2 surgeries, I read The 100 Year Lifestyle book and was able to find ways to prioritize my health and my life. I was able to make simple changes to my diet such as eliminating gluten and (artificial) sugars. I started training and competing in races including triathlons and half marathons. I also attended two ChiroMission trips, both of which were 3 weeks post-surgery. Surrounding myself with Doctors of Chiropractic that lived and taught the principle helped me see the bigger picture that I could learn from this experience and use it to teach others by providing a Lifestyle Care education. I am now 2 years cancer-free and can't wait to live to be 100 years old, healthy and on purpose! I have graduated and recently started my own Chiropractic practice in Vancouver, BC and am very excited to share The 100 Year Lifestyle with my patients and peers everywhere!

In the largest nature/nurture study that was ever done, on 44,000 pairs of twins, it was found that the primary determinates in most cases of cancer were environmental or lifestyle factors such as tobacco use, diet and exercise habits rather than the inherited disposition of their family history. The important message here if you want to live an active, healthy, quality of life for 80, 90, 100 years and beyond is… stop blaming your genes. Adjust your lifestyle and you can change the course of your history today!

Centenarian Secret

Resisting the things you know you need to change polarizes your life. This keeps you stuck. However, when you embrace change, the pieces of your life will fall naturally into place and stay there, just like the magnets.

What do you want to change? What is your Innate Intelligence screaming at you to change? Do you want to be thinner, smarter, better paid, more loved, or healthier? What will you do to attract these things with ease? It's time for a magnet flip. Trust your Innate. Let your quest for quality and not crisis motivate you if you are ready to upgrade to your ideal 100 Year-Lifestyle.

While you are in the process of thinking about what you want to change, things may look and feel difficult. Vacillating between crisis and quality-of-life motivation can keep you on an emotional roller coaster—with respect to your health, your marriage, your kids, and your finances. But, once you've made the commitment to change— and I mean *really* made it—then you will find that many of the things you have been struggling with will fall into place. Activities and choices that aren't in alignment with creating your best life will lose their appeal. Like flipping the magnet, you will begin to attract the people and resources you need to reach your greatest dreams and goals once you shift your belief about what you think you can accomplish. Whether it is health for 100 years or undying passion for your family or a hobby, you get to decide what happens, and how you respond to what happens, on your journey to a sensational century.

This resistance to change is something I observed time and again over the past quarter century, as I worked with thousands of patients, and doctors, to help them heal and optimize the quality of their lives. One of my patients was a successful stockbroker named Jim. About twice a year, Jim would come to my chiropractic office for "Crisis Care" when he was experiencing severe episodes of back pain. Each time, I would encourage him to change his life by correcting the underlying condition in his spine, rather than just slapping a "Band-Aid" on his symptoms. Jim would always respond by telling me that he knew I was right, but that he "just didn't have the time to commit to it." When I asked Jim if he had time for his current crisis, he would laugh and say, "Of course not," but he wasn't interested in changing his routine.

Over the years, the episodes would get more painful, more expensive, and more inconvenient for Jim. His spine and nervous system deteriorated over time, just like Max's. Each time Jim came in, we would talk about making the Critical Transition to Lifestyle Care and how much better it would be if he allowed quality of life to motivate his health choices instead of crisis. Finally, after years of deteriorating health and one inconvenient crisis after another, Jim committed to change. He made taking care of his spine and nervous system and spending more time with his family a priority. Two years later, he was happier and healthier than I had ever seen him. "I feel young and energetic again," he said. His business was better than ever, his marriage was better than ever, and he was playing more golf (and better golf) than ever. He was truly enjoying his best life.

Jim's quality of life was lousy when he was just thinking about changing it, but once he finally committed to making the changes he knew he needed to make and made those changes his lifestyle, he began to magnetically attract great things into his life naturally.

Life Changing Principle #2: Change Happens One Choice at Time–Think Progress, Not Perfection.

As you learn how to make the changes that will support your best life today and in the future, remember that you may not see results right away.

One of the principles of change is that the results occur over time. We "titrate" into it slowly. I've borrowed the term *titration* from the chemistry experiment most of us conducted in school. You know the one. It was the lesson where your teacher gave you a glass beaker filled with a clear liquid and a dropper with another chemical solution. You were asked to take the chemical and drop it into the beaker one drop at a time and record how many drops it took to change the liquid's color. Do you remember how nothing happened at first? You would drop, drop, drop and it would still be clear, but then suddenly, one last drop, and the liquid's color would instantly change!

In the process of chemical titration, you are determining the exact number of drops necessary to produce the desired effect or change in the solution. The question many students found themselves asking was "which drop was the most important?" Some believed it was the first drop because it began the transformation. Others thought it was the last one because that's the one where they actually saw the liquid change color. The truth is that they are all of equal importance, because without any one of them, the solution would not have changed.

This is how the results from the changes you make often appear. You have to lose one pound at a time before you finally shed 50. You have to walk a minute before you can make it a mile. Change arrives one input at a time, one choice at a time. It is an accumulation of actions that will color your life with joy or suffering—depending upon the quality of your choices.

What kind of commitment and actions do you think it will take before you start seeing the rewards of your efforts?

You can never be sure how many "drops" or acts of changed behavior it will take to get you to your desired destination. This is why you must approach change with faith and a healthy attitude— acknowledging progress without sabotaging your own success by demanding perfection. What you can be sure of, though, is this: The color and quality of your life will fade if you always choose to let crisis be your motivating force.

Now that you know it's possible to live a century or longer, how will you spend the rest of your years? What kind of drops will you add to your life each day? Will you wear out your body and mind in the first 40, 50, or 60 years, or make the most of today while you also set yourself up for decades of exciting milestone birthdays ahead? The truth is, you don't get to choose how and when you are going to die, but you can choose how you're going to live. By changing your life today and making those changes your new lifestyle, you will impact the level of health and prosperity (or suffering) you experience right now, today, and as you age.

Drop, Drop, Drop

Your titration drops affect your family members, friends and future generations. What choices are you making that will affect others?

Each choice you make will build momentum for the future while giving you confidence and enthusiasm in the present. Remember, when you choose, you are either choosing to stay on the path of your ideal 100 Year Lifestyle, or you are choosing something else. If you are going to make progress at something over the next 20, 30, or 40 years, why not make progress toward the things that you value the most. Every choice that would improve your life when you are 100 would also improve your life today.

> **Centenarian Secret**
> Your ideal 100 Year Lifestyle choices will positively impact your life today, as well as when you are 60, 70, 80, 90, or 100.

Many of us make toxic choices that limit our life. In fact, they often come disguised as rewards. For instance, have you ever reached for a cigarette as a reward at the end of a hard day or downed another dessert as an emotional pick-me-up? Were the five minutes of enjoyment worth the three days of guilt and two weeks of trying to get back on track? Your true reward comes from the self-esteem and love you give yourself when you honor yourself with each choice.

Make the rest of your life the best of your life by committing to the changes you need to make today, and then recommitting to them every day, each time you are faced with a choice. If you want to be nicotine-free, you have to make that commitment and then recommit to it every minute of every day. If you want to invest money, then you have to make that commitment and recommit to walking away from empty purchases each day. If you want to be healthy and fit, then prove it to yourself every day with each choice.

If you find yourself getting off track from your goals, it's okay. Think progress, not perfection. You can nudge yourself back on track with your next choice knowing you are in the process of building the lifestyle you can enjoy for 80, 90, 100 years and beyond.

LIFE CHANGING PRINCIPLE #3:

APPROACH CHANGE WITH YOUR IDEAL
100 YEAR LIFESTYLE IN MIND

Welcome to Life Changing Principle #3. It's time to go for the gold, whatever that means to you, as you start approaching your life with a fresh, new perspective and develop an exciting vision for the rest of your life. It is a shift that will allow you to keep your brains, your looks, your possessions, and your mojo as you age. It is a shift that will allow you to live your ideal 100 Year Lifestyle without compromise. It is time to draw a line in the sand and declare that the balance of your life will be the most fun, exciting, and fulfilling times you have ever experienced. You can use your M-PYR to build your empire.

A few years ago, I had a patient who needed to lose weight. Bill was a former athlete but he had committed so much time to his marriage, raising his kids, and working that his health had declined slowly over time. He worked hard at getting rid of his extra weight, but it never seemed to stay off. As he "dieted", he constantly focused on what he could not have. He felt very restricted and disliked the taste of the low-fat, unhealthy substitutes he was consuming. The process was a slow and unsatisfying rollercoaster. I knew he needed and wanted to change.

One day, I sat Bill down and helped him see how losing weight wasn't about *losing* anything at all. I explained that his choice to trim down meant he was really *gaining* muscle, energy, and self-esteem. He was building a stronger heart and overall health. His goals seemed more attainable when he changed his focus. He approached his new nutrition and lifestyle habits not from a belief that he was losing something, but from a belief that he was gaining a life that he could really be excited about. So he made the changes he knew he needed to make, and two weeks later he came in for his chiropractic adjustment wearing exercise clothes, looking "fast and fit," and he said he was feeling younger than he had felt in 25 years.

Just as change that focuses on "loss" can be hard to sustain, so is change that results in lateral movement. One of my colleagues was struggling in her practice and decided to close up shop and reopen in a different town. She changed her location, but she never expanded her skill set or changed how she practiced. Her new practice ended up just like the old one—with the same old problems as the ones she tried to leave behind.

She was not able to create a better practice because her focus was not in the right place. She made a sideways move that caused a superficial shift and the same stressful result. Instead, she might have looked at how the health care industry was changing, how to improve the quality of her care, or how the needs of her patients were evolving. You see this happen with people again and again—not just professionally, but even in terms of their relationships. People make knee-jerk actions without slowing down and taking time to consider the true nature of their situation. In the case of my colleague, she approached change not with her ideal 100 Year Lifestyle in mind, but with the idea of escaping the mistakes she had made in her old location. It was an approach that kept her stuck in her old destructive patterns.

Centenarian Secret

Approaching change with your ideal 100 Year Lifestyle in mind is the key to creating lasting results. This is how you will optimize the quality and quantity of your life. It is the only focus that will keep you consistently motivated during your "titration" process—as you get from where you are to where you want to be.

With this knowledge, you now have the opportunity to make the changes that will lead you toward an incredible 100 Year Lifestyle. You may be wondering where to start. What are the means for getting to this end? How much money will you want? How will you nurture your marriage and other relationships over this extended period of time?

The questions I've developed for you at the end of this chapter will help you begin to personalize and prioritize your plan. First, you need to get in touch with what you really want and deserve. This can sometimes be challenging, particularly when it is out of step with the values of your family or peer group. However, if that's the case, you may have been more of a follower than a leader and it's time to take back the reins. Now is your time to step up and take charge. You'll soon see that you will not only start creating positive change in your own life, but also in the lives of people around you. You'll be a healthy influence. Expect some relationships to deepen and some to be strained or fall away. You will open the door to magnetically attracting support for your 100 Year Lifestyle from all kinds of unexpected people, places and resources. As you begin to customize your vision, don't settle. Dare yourself. Stretch yourself. Go for the goal that burns brightest in your gut.

Expect progress—not perfection—as you embark on this new journey that I will guide you on throughout this book, on our website at www.100yearlifestyle.com, our Facebook Fan Page at www.facebook.com/100yearlifestyle and The 100 Year Lifestyle YouTube channel. Although you don't have complete control over how long you'll live, you've got control over your attitude and your choices that impact the quality of those years. Assume you are here for a reason. Spend your days discovering that reason. Relax into the ebb and flow of life. Trust yourself, your Innate Intelligence, and begin to connect with your core like never before. Find the meaning and opportunity in everything. When you do that, the length of your life doesn't matter anyway. The ultimate question will be whether you fulfilled your purpose and lived your life to the fullest and without regret.

In the chapters ahead, you'll customize your 100 Year Lifestyle. You'll learn how to live healthier, longer, become wiser, optimize your environment, eliminate stress, and establish routines, relationships, and learning patterns that will support you in that lifestyle. You will capitalize on time (since you are going to have so much more of it than you thought), expand your income, and build a compass for lasting purpose.

Now let's get specific and personal.

LIVE LONG AND STRONG

In each of the following areas, write in the changes you want to make with your ideal 100 Year Lifestyle in mind:
- Your health?
- Your environment?
- Your schedule?
- Your finances?
- Your relationships?
- Your career?
- How you spend your free time?
- How you use your talents?
- How you manage stress?
- The way you treat people or how you allow them to treat you?
- The way you think about your past?
- The way you approach your future?

Make these changes your lifestyle.

Choose up to three areas that are the most important to you. Commit to change. Then, be prepared to recommit to those changes every time you are faced with a choice.

Remember, staying the same and compromising yourself will be harder than just making the change. Your hesitation is what keeps you on the emotional and results roller coaster. Once you commit, all of that emotional energy can be directed to your highest values. Whether it's exercising more, eating healthier, or managing your time and money better—make choices with your 100 Year Lifestyle in mind. You will improve your life today and improve your life tomorrow while you balance your desire for immediate gratification with your long-term desires. Always keep in mind the present and future that you want to experience—this will ensure that the quality of your years keeps pace with the quantity.

It's time to declare your vision for the next phase of your life. What would you like your next decade to be like? Whether you live to 70, 80, 90, or 100-plus, the choices you make today will define the depth and breadth of what you experience tomorrow.

Don't worry about whether you'll have the strength and discipline to follow through on your 100 Year Lifestyle. One day at a time, one choice at a time, we'll do it together and God-willing, enjoy a sensational century.

Turn the page now and find the energy to change with the excitement of knowing you are just getting started. The fun has just begun.

THE 100 YEAR LIFESTYLE
ACTION PLAN FOR LASTING CHANGE

1. *Take Advantage of the Advanced Notice.* Calculate your M-PYR. Calculate your family's M-PYR. Listen to the advanced notice your parents and grandparents are giving you about how long you can and probably will live. Make life choices for the long haul. Start planning your 100 Year Lifestyle today, so you can experience a life of lasting health, wealth, prosperity, partnership, and purpose as you age. Your minimum potential years remaining are not your maximum.

2. *Put the Three Life-Changing Principles to Work for You.* These principles represent the simple truth about change that can keep you consistently committed to the changes you know you want and need to make.

3. *Change Is Easy—Thinking about Change Is Hard.* Change happens one choice at a time. Think progress, not perfection. Approach change with your ideal 100 Year Lifestyle in mind.

4. *Choose Quality-of-Life Motivation—Not Crisis Motivation.* Allowing crisis to motivate you to change keeps you in your old patterns and issues. Choose quality of life motivation over the crisis approach to change. That way, you'll avoid many painful, unnecessary detours along the way.

5. *Choose Up to Three Areas to Change.* What are the priority areas of your life you want to change? Whether it's your health, your finances, your work, or relationships, choose up to three and start titrating change into them today. Lasting change is easy when you allow yourself to build momentum.

6. *Approach Change with Your Ideal 100 Year Lifestyle in Mind.* Choose your focus. Your best life choices are ones that will positively impact your life both today and when you are 60, 70, 80, 90, or 100. This focus will give you a foundation of clear and lasting commitment to becoming the best you.

7. *The Rest of Your Life Can Be the Best of Your Life.* Dare yourself! Make it a sensational century. Live and leave your best life legacy as you learn how to live longer, healthier, and wiser than any other generation in history.

PART 2

Enjoying Youthful Energy at Every Age

Wherever you focus your energy, that's where it goes.

CHAPTER 3

FINDING THE ENERGY TO CHANGE YOUR LIFE

If you're excited to start living The 100 Year Lifestyle but aren't sure you've got the energy for it, I've got some exciting news for you. It's not your age that's exhausting you. It is how you choose to use your energy that either wears you out or wakes you up. Wherever you focus your energy, that's where it goes.

If your life is anything like mine, you probably operate at a fast pace. In fact, thinking about changing your schedule or making commitments may seem even more exhausting than keeping up with your current routine. That's why so many of us unintentionally wait for a crisis to create the extra energy we need to justify changing our lives. We don't intend to stay in the status quo or rob ourselves of our health, hopes and dreams. Yet, somehow we end up on autopilot.

Why we do it is unique to each of us. Some of us lack drive. Some of us love the familiar. Maybe we are comfortable. The reasons really aren't that important. The truth is that change is a high-energy investment that appreciates over time and the good news is that your energy to change already exists. The question is where have you been spending it?

I was recently working with a doctor who was unhappy with his practice. He wanted to make a change. Managed care had hurt his profitability. His practice felt more like a burden than a joy.

Though he was an excellent healer, he was losing the passion he once had for his work. When I began suggesting what he could do to make his vocation fun and exciting again, I was shocked by his reaction. He began to argue with me, insisting that it wasn't possible. He focused on why he couldn't make the changes he knew he needed to make.

His face got red. His posture became defensive. There was an edge in his voice. The amount of energy he expended to defend why he couldn't change was incredible. He ran down a list of at least ten different reasons why things had to stay the same. Five minutes into the conversation, I felt more like I was in a courtroom with a defense attorney rather than a coaching session. He had built a tremendous case against himself, defending why he couldn't change. I was listening to some of the negative chatter that played inside his head, day after day. The chatter was, in large part, unconscious.

A few days later, I was talking with a patient who was a very successful entrepreneur. Her all work, no play routine was taking a toll on her health and her family. She was exhausted. Her back hurt, and her level of stress was off the charts. When I suggested she take some time for herself, she began to argue with me, listing the reasons why she couldn't. Her clients wouldn't like it, she told me. Her cell phone interrupted our conversation several times and we had to constantly start over again. It was tiring just watching her. This woman is a great salesperson and she could sell anything to anybody. Her challenge was that she had sold herself on the fact that she couldn't change. And she was wasting a lot of energy in the process. No wonder she was stuck and exhausted.

I asked these two people, who were having trouble finding the energy to change, the same question that I am about to ask you:

WHOSE SIDE ARE YOU ON, ANYWAY?

They soon discovered, as you will too, that one of the places where the energy to change springs from is the decision to stop defending why you can't change. What would happen if you started to build a case for why you can live your ideal 100 Year Lifestyle, instead of investing your energy in arguing why you can't? After all, remember your M-PYR? You may have a minimum of 40, 50, 60 or even 70 more years ahead of you. Your newfound energy will come from the same place it comes from now, only you will use it differently. You will use it to support, encourage, and take action to make the rest of your life the best. Your energy level would skyrocket.

HOW TO MASTER CHANGE

Remember Life Changing Principle #1: *Change is easy. Thinking about it is hard.* In the long run, staying the same often requires more energy than changing. When you don't make the changes you know you need to make, your energy is wasted on survival, boredom, anger, and frustration—that creates stress, worry, anxiety, and other energy-draining emotions. When you recognize it, you can consciously begin to change the way you expend your energy which can miraculously restore your enthusiasm, health, success, and vigor.

What would you do if you were to suffer from a disability? Would you stay in the safety of your wheelchair or tackle the world and embrace your life? Would you play the victim and defend your limitations with all your energy or would you build the case for why you can overcome them, be healthy, and live your unique 100 Year Lifestyle?

Living The 100 Year Lifestyle: No Excuses

25-year-old Kyle Maynard knows what I'm talking about.

You may have seen Kyle on *ESPN*, *Oprah*, in *USA Today*, or in one of the many other magazines that have featured his story. Kyle was born without full limbs. Standing only two and a half feet tall and weighing 123 pounds, this courageous young athlete chose to join his school wrestling team at the age of 11.

Most people thought what he was attempting to do the impossible. But his parents supported his determination to learn the sport. Kyle, who walks and runs on all fours, spent hours practicing each day. But his first 35 matches were losses.

As a sophomore and junior, Kyle finally titrated into winning. By his senior year, his record of 35-16 placed him in the top 3 in Georgia and the top 12 in the nationals. A broken nose is all that kept him from being named All American in 2004. Today, Kyle is a best-selling author of the book *No Excuses*, an entrepreneur and a mighty motivational speaker.

How has he overpowered his wrestling opponents? He triumphs because, believe it or not, his challengers see him as having the advantage. His opponents believe Kyle's small stature makes him swifter and stronger than they are. What an irony that someone with congenitally amputated arms and legs could have the upper hand!

What an honor it was for me to provide Kyle with the performance-based chiropractic care that helped him set a world record in his weight class. There are no limits when there is no interference and no excuses! Kyle recently opened a new gym called CrossFit No Excuses and in 2012 he took his 'no excuses' attitude to Tanzania and climbed the majestic 20,000 foot Mt. Kilimanjaro.

Many of us use "what's missing" in our lives as the reason for why we can't change or why we can't reach our goals. "Instead of telling people what I am going to try to do, I just go out and do it," says Kyle. "Once they see it, then they believe it can be done."

One of the reasons thinking about change (Life Changing Principle #1) is so hard is that the indecision and uncertainty eats up a lot of your Innate energy. Many of us fear change because we are afraid of how other people will react. Often, it seems easier to stay where we are. But when you choose change and commit to it, you'll find in time that your own certainty and confidence surpasses those fears and doubts and gets you moving forward. You begin to magnetically attract support as the people around you realize that you are serious and committed to your new life.

As you saw with Kyle, this can happen slowly over time or it can happen the instant you truly decide without looking back.

Centenarian Secret

Great things happen when you have the wherewithal to stick to your commitments and follow through. You find yourself respected by people you respect. You create a life story that inspires other people. You show other people what is possible. Have the grit to see it through. Go for your ideal 100 Year Lifestyle. If not now, when? How many more decades will you compromise yourself and what you know Innately is right for you?

Quite often, the reasons why you think you can't change are the reasons why you can, should, and must. If you think you can't find the time to exercise because you've got to take the kids to school, cook dinner, and pay the bills, then that's the reason why you should. If you don't, you are shorting both yourself and your family by giving them a partial you—someone who is exhausted, edgy, and resentful all the time.

CHANGE HAPPENS ONE CHOICE AT A TIME

Right now, I would like you to think of one thing you would like to change. For example, maybe you are suffering from a health problem and you need to make your health your top priority. Maybe you just retired from a position you held for 25 years and you are looking for something new to which you can commit. Maybe you are looking to get into a relationship. No matter what type of change you may be contemplating, ask yourself these questions:

What are my most important values?

Who are the people in my life who can support me in reaching my goals?

What experiences and skills do I already have that can get me where I want to go?

From here, start to design and take action on your plan.

Living The 100 Year Lifestyle: Chanda Hinton

Chanda Hinton is the founder of The Chanda Plan Foundation. When she was 9 years old, she suffered a serious, life-threatening injury that left her partially paralyzed and forced to learn a new way of living. Chanda's interest in alternative health care started in 2003. Her spinal cord injury had compromised her health to the degree that her weight had dropped to 59 pounds, she had chronic pain and her immune system had depleted to a dangerous level leading to 911 emergency care and numerous doctor visits. Her increased intake of prescription drugs was alarming and she knew she was on a destructive path. Chanda and her sister decided to take the actions they discussed regarding her participation in holistic healing. In the following months Chanda's choice to pursue health care providers such as chiropractors and acupuncturists who would promote healing by relieving the stress on her structure, spine and nervous system enabled her to gain weight and become almost pain free. In addition, her endurance, strength and movement increased dramatically.

Most insurance that people with disabilities have for healthcare and homecare expenses created by their disability will not fund alternative treatments. Through a concerted outreach effort, Chanda developed a team of healers that provided her care for zero cost. Due to her once unimaginable improvements, Chanda is dedicated to having this care accessible to others through her foundation. She says, "When you are in good health, fulfilling the things you are passionate about seems limitless." Consider making a donation at www.thechandaplanfoundation.org

Sure, becoming healthy when you have been sick can be a challenge and require a lot of focus. Changing your health habits from Crisis Care to Lifestyle Care requires awareness, discipline and follow-through. Starting a revenue-generating business on a shoe string budget can be complicated. Opening up your heart to an intimate relationship can be scary. Yes, all these things are very possible and achievable when you commit to change, then make one choice at a time with your ideal 100 Year Lifestyle in mind.

As you read through the rest of this book, you'll find the tools and strategies to help you succeed. Your mind and body will become stocked with the energy and power to make these changes you know you need to make. Understand, though, that to create change, *you* will need to change. You must BE different and you must start doing things differently. You can't always go with the flow—but to change you have to let go.

ENERGY DRAINERS VERSUS ENERGY ENHANCERS

Your energy is one of your most valuable resources, so be selective about how and where you focus it. Don't waste a drop. Even though high-energy human potential is your natural state, you only have so much in a given day. Stress and other distractions can easily deplete this gift if you allow them to drain you. Every thought, action and decision you make regarding your health, relationships, business, exercise, diet, emotional reactions, and achievements either positively or negatively impacts your energy.

According to the laws of physics, energy can neither be created nor destroyed. This rule, known as the Law of Conservation, says that there is a constant and finite amount of energy in the world. This energy can be converted, however, to produce the outcomes you desire.

This is what happens when we bounce a ball. When you hold a ball above the ground, it has potential energy to fall. When you release the ball, and it begins to move, the energy becomes kinetic. Kinetic energy changes the ball's momentum. Electrical energy from a battery can be converted into mechanical energy to move your car. A small amount of nuclear energy can light the night sky across an entire city.

Have you ever noticed how when you're on fire about a project, your energy soars in much the same way? When you are committed to the things that matter to you, you connect with your Innate energy and fuel your efforts with a type of kinetic energy that gives you the momentum to transform your life.

You can feel younger every day with your current energy supply if you are willing to redistribute the way you choose to use it. Everyday choices, thoughts and habits will either support or undermine your Innate energy. Choose wisely. Do this by distancing yourself from people or situations that deplete you. Stop overreacting. Get up off the couch. For me, drinking too much caffeine and not exercising drains my energy. Going for walks and spending time with my wife and children enhances it.

Now is the time to become your own personal energy leader. You will immediately feel younger and healthier than you have in a long time—regardless of your age. After all, High Energy Human Potential is your natural state. How you choose to use your energy is up to you.

When you master your own energy, you will sustain that high state of energy and avoid radical highs and lows. Like programming your home to a comfortable temperature so that the air conditioner turns on when it gets too hot or the heat turns on when it's too cold, you can program your own energy level for consistently high output.

TAKE A PERSONAL ENERGY INVENTORY

Energy drainers and energy enhancers are very personal so it is critical that you listen to your Innate Intelligence. What may be an energy drainer for one person may be an energy enhancer for another. I remember participating in a board meeting where the topic was the bylaws of the organization. The lawyers in the group were passionately debating every word. In the thick of it, my colleague grinned at me and said, "I love this." What was energizing for him was exhausting and draining for me. I kept looking at my watch, counting the seconds as I felt the energy being zapped from my body, while he kept leaping back into the conversation and picking up steam.

Shopping is another activity that energizes some and depletes others. Some people just love "the hunt" and they are captivated by everything that is shiny and new. Others are more focused on the crowds, rude salespeople, and the challenge of tracking down what they really need. However, there are many activities that universally charge us up or deplete us. Most people are energized by quality time with family and friends, or reading a good book. On the other hand, some universal energy drainers include overworking, overeating, drinking too much alcohol and taking drugs.

Once you take your Personal Energy Inventory, you can consciously begin to make choices that support your high-energy 100 Year Lifestyle. Eliminate the things that drain you. Focus on the things that energize you. When you do this, you will find that you Innately have the resources you need to change your life. In fact, not making the change is an energy drainer. The commitment to change ignites a spark for instant energy. Recommitting to that change with every choice provides you with a continual feed. For example, if you detest shopping in stores, hire someone to shop for you, or consider shopping online. These days, you can buy most everything you need this way. And doing so frees up time to pursue a potential business idea, play with your children or grandchildren, or plan a special occasion with your spouse.

Here is a sample list of activities that will measure how well you are using your potential energy. It will help you identify the quality of the choices you are making as they relate to your energy, and whether they are helping or hurting you. Each action is either a credit or debit toward your energy bank.

Use your answers to help you shift your energy to live your ideal 100 Year Lifestyle.

LIVE LONG AND STRONG
Check off the statements below that apply to you.
My Energy Enhancers:
- ☐ Speaking my truth
- ☐ Quality time with kids
- ☐ Being honest
- ☐ Following through
- ☐ Reading good books
- ☐ Keeping promises to myself
- ☐ Being grateful
- ☐ Prayer
- ☐ Eating healthy
- ☐ Getting my chiropractic adjustments
- ☐ Supplementing my diet
- ☐ Date night with spouse
- ☐ Quality time with friends
- ☐ Focusing on the positive
- ☐ Having faith
- ☐ Expressing gratitude
- ☐ Standing up for myself
- ☐ Staying on task
- ☐ Letting go of the things that are out of my control
- ☐ Taking action on my goals
- ☐ Making time to exercise
- ☐ Good posture
- ☐ Massages
- ☐ Saving money
- ☐ Being involved in things I believe in
- ☐ Celebrating special occasions

My Energy Drainers:
- ☐ Sugar
- ☐ Caffeine
- ☐ Not exercising
- ☐ Arguing with my spouse
- ☐ Stress
- ☐ Spinal Subluxations
- ☐ Drama
- ☐ Interruptions
- ☐ Being overweight
- ☐ Over-scheduling my day
- ☐ Saying yes when I mean no
- ☐ Overworking
- ☐ Not taking Play Time
- ☐ Taking abuse
- ☐ Worry
- ☐ Slouching
- ☐ Overanalyzing
- ☐ Trying to change other people
- ☐ Being a people pleaser
- ☐ Stressing out
- ☐ Mindless television
- ☐ Not having a purpose
- ☐ Not completing things that I start

On what types of activities do you spend most of your time? Do you tend to do things that fuel you? Or do you find that most of your time is spent on activities that deplete you? Your Personal Energy Inventory is a reality check on where your energy is being distributed. I don't want you to perceive it as a list of problems, or a way to defend why things are the way they are. Instead, it is a way to raise your awareness about where all your energy is going and how to get it flowing back into your life.

Every energy drainer has an energy enhancer that can take its place. You just have to train yourself to make that choice. Very often, we find the energy to change by saying no to the activities, habits, and patterns that drain us. Not doing can be just as important as doing.

How you think can also be an energy drainer or an energy enhancer. If worry is a big energy drain for you, try turning your worry into faith. Recently, after going through this exercise with one of my clients, she told me that over the last 30 years of her adult life, she worried all the time. "Nothing that I ever worried about ever happened, but it took so much of my energy. I have so much energy now, sometimes I feel like I don't even need to sleep." Turning worry into faith and strengthening your ability to accept things you cannot change will free up a tremendous amount of your energy. One great saying to help you let go is the Serenity Prayer: "God give me the serenity to accept the things I cannot change, the courage to change the things I can, and the wisdom to know the difference." This is a great mantra if one of your energy leaks is trying to control other people.

After all, worry never made a deposit into a bank account, healed a disease, or changed the weather. Converting worry into an energy-enhancing attitude can free you to direct your energy toward powering change. As you feel your energy grow, it will enhance your creative spirit and set you on the path that will bring you all of the answers and resources to drive your fun, exciting, adventurous 100 Year Lifestyle. You will no longer dread the changes you know you need to make and you will take action. You might consider reading a book on a subject you are passionate about, scheduling a trip that you have always wanted to take, making an appointment with your chiropractor, nutritionist, or personal trainer or decide to let go of your need to control. It's your list. Trust your Innate to know what is best for you.

YOUR PERSONAL ENERGY INVENTORY

On the left side of this box, list your most draining personal energy drainers. On the right side of this box, list your most enhancing energy enhancers. Add to this list every day as you go through your day and experience things that wear you down or inspire your energy. Once your list is complete, live on the right side of this box and sustain youthful energy regardless of your age.

Energy Drainers

_____

_____

_____

_____

_____

_____

_____

Energy Enhancers

_____

_____

_____

_____

_____

_____

_____

EMPLOY ENERGY ENHANCERS

Theoretically, we watch television or surf the internet to entertain ourselves. But all too often the television, computer or smart phone becomes an uncomfortable, addictive diversion from an exhausting workday, a rude salesclerk, or a family problem. The latter makes these technologies an energy drainer. After dinner, rather than settle in with two scoops of ice cream and the remote, you might try going for a power walk, reading, Pilates, or gardening. You will feel incredible doing energy enhancing activities like this and you will sleep better. As a result, you will feel more energized the next day.

Taking a sauna, doing yoga, and drinking a lot of water are also excellent ways to set up a restorative sleep. Other energy-enhancing ideas include walking with neighbors and inviting friends over. You know what energizes and fills you with positive energy better than anyone else. Seek out and fill your life with these choices, and make this your lifestyle. Don't be afraid to vary them and try new things—mixing them up is a great way to optimize their benefits and keep things fresh.

It's time to optimize your Innate energy and make High Energy Human Potential your natural state by saying "no" to the attitudes and actions that drain you and "yes" to the energy enhancers that fuel you. This is how you will generate the currency to power your ideal 100 Year Lifestyle.

CHAPTER 4

HABITS THAT OPTIMIZE YOUR PERSONAL ENERGY

The energy drainers and energy enhancers that are a part of your personality and everyday life make up your habits or Dominant Energy Patterns (DEPs). These habit patterns can be conscious or unconscious. Become aware of them and you can train yourself to shift into a higher gear in an instant.

If you are content with your current energy level and you can see 100 years of exciting living ahead of you, then congratulations. The rest of this book will give you the tools and resources you need to make the most of your solid foundation. If not, you can choose to change your habit patterns and redefine yourself by identifying your current DEP and consciously choosing a new one, one that will support your ideal 100 Year Lifestyle.

In the movie *Super Size Me*, Morgan Spurlock went from a health nut to fast-food junkie for 30 days to see how this shift in eating patterns would affect his life. He also stopped exercising. Prior to his experiment, he was in excellent health. It was amazing what 30 days of fast-food living did to him. His weight ballooned, his cholesterol zoomed, and his liver was showing signs of distress. We should thank Morgan for showing us that, when you alter your patterns, you alter your life. Morgan also demonstrated that when you change your patterns back, your body heals and becomes healthy again. In other words, like it or not, you become your Dominant Energy Pattern.

What are your patterns? Really think about it. Your patterns include how you think, what you eat, where you shop, what you watch on TV, who you hang around with, the books you read, and more. As a society, we label people by their patterns. We admire "workaholics" and abhor "losers." Some of us are "night owls" and others are "morning persons." We've been on dates with "party animals," "bookworms," and "geeks." We size up other people by their patterns, but rarely do we do so with ourselves.

Is your Dominant Energy Pattern aligned with your potential?

You can measure your day-to-day connection with your Dominant Energy Pattern by the intensity of your energy level. Consistently sustaining high energy each day is usually a pretty good indicator that you are operating at your highest level of human potential and your pattern probably supports this. It means you have succeeded in keeping the drama out of your day, avoided second-guessing yourself, and interacted with others from a place of personal integrity. This fuels each hour with purpose. Just the opposite is true if you find yourself constantly scrambling to get by. You can, through the three life-changing principles, permanently re-create your Dominant Energy Pattern to fuel the rest of your life.

The following are the five DEPs that shape your life—whether you are aware of it or not. Do you know which pattern you are in right now?

1. Destructive patterns
2. Survival patterns
3. Complacency patterns

4. Comfort patterns

5. Human potential patterns

DEP #1: DESTRUCTIVE PATTERNS

If you're stuck in a destructive energy pattern, you are probably overspending, overeating, overdrinking, overmedicating, overworking, oversleeping, or overdoing something. You know what it is. Destructive patterns are dangerous because they often end up in addictions, thoughts or feelings that can spin your life out of control. It is a pattern usually comprised of repeated behaviors that unconsciously deteriorate your quality of life.

Maybe the first time you chose the actions related to these patterns, you thought about it before you did it. For instance, the first pain pill, diet pill or first bite of sugar might have been conscious, but the second, fifth, and tenth were not. Now these patterns occur so spontaneously that you don't even think about them anymore. Most of us feel better after we buy something, but if you hate yourself after the bill comes because you don't have enough money to pay it, it has become a destructive pattern. If you were to truly, consciously choose to take this action consciously right now, would it be your first, second or even third choice? If not, this action may be part of a destructive pattern for you.

Rather than fueling your Innate energy, these actions typically leave you empty inside. Some people who are living in a chronic destructive energy pattern can often point to a place on their body where they feel like an "empty well" exists. It may be a hollow pressure in the chest around the heart or lungs or some other physical manifestation of the emotional pain and emptiness caused by long-term destructive energy patterns.

We all feel this hole in our lives and feel it intensely at one time or another. It is a hole that we want to close but often don't know how. Destructive energy patterns may give you a spike of energy in the beginning, but usually, they are followed by an energy crash filled with anger, resentment, or low self-esteem. They end up widening the hollow opening rather than closing it, which can actually make the pain more intense.

This seemingly bottomless pit gets larger when it is fed with destructive patterns such as smoking, drinking, prescription and non-prescription drugs, laziness, procrastination, overeating, and erroneous thinking. It also feeds on negative emotions like blame, anger, hopelessness, and hate. How do you reverse the process if you have already arrived at a place where you feel empty, blank, or lost as a result of your choices that are destructive to your long-term well-being? How do you close the hole and refocus your energy? The hole shrinks as you speak and live your truth. It will shrink as you align your actions with your highest vision of yourself one choice at a time, as with Life Changing Principle #2: Change comes one choice at a time; think progress not perfection. Every time you make a choice that leads to progress, the hole will feel a little smaller. When you don't, you may get a temporary high followed by a widening of the hole and an empty, hollow feeling inside.

Destructive energy patterns involve compromising yourself and not keeping your commitments to yourself. On both a subconscious and a conscious level, your body knows and you know what level of destruction you are causing. Don't ignore the evidence, which causes you to wake up to a much bigger problem down the road.

Don't Be An Ostrich

Have you ever seen a picture of an ostrich with its head buried in the sand? This is one of the funniest scenes in nature and is a great metaphor to describe individuals who have a Crisis Care mentality about their health. This means that they only take care of themselves when they get sick, diagnosed with a disease or are in excruciating pain. This is not a good idea.

If you want to live an active, healthy long life, it's time to redefine crisis. Here are early signs that you or your loved ones are in crisis or are headed for one.

1.   You take over the counter drugs on a monthly basis
2.   You have taken prescription drugs consistently for more than three months
3.   You have altered your life due to a health concern
4.   You constantly try to pop your neck and back or are fidgety
5.   You cannot or do not exercise
6.   You take medication to offset the side effects of other medications
7.   You experience irregular sleep patterns
8.   You are susceptible to colds and the flu
9.   You often say things like "I don't feel right." Or, "I need to take a pill."
10. You have difficulty standing or sitting up straight.

Many seniors and centenarians are suffering the consequences of their "If it ain't broke, don't fix it" ostrich-like attitudes. We are getting the advance notice that our parents and grandparents never received. The principles of The 100 Year Lifestyle will help you think differently about your health and pull your head out of the sand.

Destructive energy patterns can be seen in thinking, eating, drinking, taking medication, working, spending, relationships, and more. Here are a few examples:

- Destructive thinking patterns can be characterized by negative self-talk, personal put downs, pessimism, closed mindedness, hopeless attitude. These thoughts that you have about yourself are not true. They are not real. They are only your current thoughts which you can change right now if you become aware of them and are willing to change them. Create a Personal Affirmation that you can rely on in times of stress that reinforces the positive. Make this a habit and your thinking will change.

- Destructive eating patterns can be characterized by automatic or emotional eating and a failure to taste your food when you eat it. You should eat to fuel your body. And you should enjoy your food while you are eating it. Don't eat food out of habit or to alleviate stress.

- Destructive eating patterns also include eating foods that you know are not good for you. Good nutrition is one of our most powerful self-care choices you can make to improve your health, increase your energy and change your pattern. Healthy eating patterns include reading about and choosing to eat foods that are good for you at each meal, and as a part of your 100 Year Lifestyle.

- Smartphones, ipads and other mobile devices may be the latest technology craze, but they are not good for you if you are addicted to them. You should not be plugged into technology around the clock. You have a destructive work pattern when you become stressed by not having immediate access to e-mail, a cell phone, or a computer or you feel that you must be doing something professionally, all the time, and you push the rest of your life away. You are in this pattern if your family and friends frequently refer to you as a workaholic. This type of pattern can take a toll—not only on your health but also on your most important relationships.

- You have destructive relationship patterns when you attract relationships that are controlling, empty, or abusive. Healthy relationships have a good balance of giving and receiving. They nurture you, make you happy, and give you a sense of support. They meet your social and emotional needs.

- Destructive relationship patterns are unsupportive. You can discern the difference between productive and destructive relationships by how you feel after spending time with someone. Avoid people and situations that inflict pain, and if you must be around these people, just don't give them your energy and certainly don't have the unrealistic expectation that they will fill you up emotionally. Going to these people for support is like going to an empty well for water. They will not quench your thirst.

THE MIDSTREAM CATCH

The Midstream Catch will stop you in the middle of a Destructive pattern, or any pattern for that matter, and give you the freedom to make a new, conscious choice in the present moment. The Midstream Catch is simple, but it is not always easy. Here are three simple steps to the Midstream Catch:

1. Become conscious and aware that you are in a Destructive pattern

2. Mentally and Physically "Stop" yourself from continuing destructive patterns in the present moment

3. Make a new choice that supports your best you

The Midstream Catch sounds simple, but it is not always easy, especially if you are addicted to your Destructive pattern. There is no shortcut to this process when it comes to changing your life. Initially you may find that you have to go through this process 1,000 times a day. Then, as time goes on, you may only need to catch yourself 50, 10 or 2 times a day. Eventually it may only be one time a week, a month or a year. Stay committed to the process and you will wake up one day and realize that you are living your ideal 100 Year Lifestyle.

DEP #2: SURVIVAL PATTERNS

If you're stuck in a survival pattern, everything is a struggle—from paying your bills to getting to work on time. You always seem to be just one step ahead of disaster. Somehow, however, you generally get by—but without a penny or a second to spare. When you live this type of life, you are fueled by adrenaline. You use stress to get things done. Some people are even addicted to stress. After all, it's a rush. It may even make you feel very important—for a little while. For some people, it even speeds up their metabolism.

You are in a survival pattern when stress has become normal to you. In fact, when you step back and observe your behavior, you'll find that you actually seek out more stressful experiences. You are late to the meeting—again. You tend to procrastinate and use imminent deadlines to get you motivated. You live right on the edge—all the time. You need the rush. People caught up in survival patterns sometimes refer to themselves as "tornadoes" and the like—they are whirling masses of energy.

Centenarian Secret

Although living with constant stress is common in today's world, this is not a way to live a sensational century. You might not even make it to 60 or 70. Eventually the roller coaster catches up to you and the chronic stress has a myriad of negative consequences. For one thing, it can eventually cause you to "crash." It's bad for your looks. And longevity experts have now shown that this chronic stress can shorten your life and precipitate obesity.

People caught up in survival patterns are generally well intentioned but shortsighted. They struggle to prioritize and figure out what really matters. Every ounce of energy is spent chasing your tail. For example, when a person's physical or financial health is out of balance, it dominates the expenditure of time and money. Priorities like buying your spouse a gift, traveling to see family, or planning a vacation take a back seat.

The good news is that if you are currently in a survival pattern, your commitment to healing will positively impact every area of your life. To escape a survival pattern, remember The Midstream Catch. You must *stop* and realize what you are doing. Catch yourself in the middle, become aware, and make an energy-enhancing choice. You must learn to take time-outs and view the bigger picture, build your reserves, and break the cycle. In some cases, you must reset your internal barometer while you establish a new human potential pattern.

If a stressful job or relationship has unconsciously moved you into this pattern, you must decide if it is worth it. Living a life in constant disarray is not a way to thrive or grow. Once you have removed the stressor, you can change your thinking. If the stressor is out of your control, change your thoughts about it. Plan long-term, set boundaries, and avoid constantly putting yourself into situations that will cause you more stress. Focus on building back your reserves and stop the crisis motivation. To escape a survival pattern, take control of your thoughts, actions and life by making different choices that support the vision of your ideal 100 Year Lifestyle, keeping in mind Life Changing Principle #3. Make your future so compelling that you are willing, with each choice in the present, to shift gears with The Midstream Catch.

DEP #3: COMPLACENCY PATTERNS

You've got things together and are getting by without worrying about survival. In a complacency pattern, life isn't a struggle, but it's nothing to write home about either. In this pattern, there is an underlying sense of boredom and laziness. There is no passion. You've resigned yourself to a life of mediocrity.

There is nothing wrong with complacency on occasion. However as a lifestyle, it is boring and will eventually erode your self-esteem and personal confidence. Before you know it, you look in the mirror with disappointment, wondering what ever happened to the flame. The truth is, you can't be mediocre and enjoy a sensational century at the same time. You have to choose. Have you resigned yourself to a ho-hum way of life? Do you really want the next 30 to 50 years to stay on this path? It is one thing to be complacent for a week, but for the rest of your life?

Many people become complacent because they don't believe their efforts will matter. They feel like they have already accomplished what they can and there is not enough time left for them to start a new career, relationship, improve their health, or become wealthy. This pattern will hit home for you if on some level you have given up on your goals. Your actions have no purpose. It's a pattern synonymous with settling, and a why-bother kind of attitude. One of the many challenges of complacency is that you tend to get out of balance with giving and receiving in your relationships.

I've worked with many patients who passionately looked forward to retiring so they could play golf all the time. Once they retired, however, they played so much golf that they didn't enjoy the game anymore. One woman in particular got so bored and disgusted with the game that a year after retiring she sold her clubs and went back to work.

There's no passion with complacency. It can make you feel tired and look older than you actually are. Setting new goals and taking action on them will re-energize you. Now that you realize you will probably have more time to accomplish all that you've wanted to achieve, why not step things up a notch and embrace your 100 Year Lifestyle? Begin to set new goals for yourself and start to make them happen. After all, knowing that you may live longer than you ever thought will enable you to start fresh with a lifetime of experience under your belt.

- If you have grown complacent at work, get back in the game. Start making things happen. Make sure that your superiors recognize your contribution. Instead of saying, "It was nothing" when you are complimented on a project, say, "Thank you for recognizing my role. It was a challenge to bring all the departments together to execute a successful program. But it was very rewarding and I'm very happy to contribute."

- Document your achievements. Begin managing your career as if you were climbing the ladder of success and build upon your wins. Utilize your documented achievements at annual reviews to ask for a pay raise or see a new job. Discuss your achievements over the past year with a focus on your results. Show your value to your employer's bottom line.

- When you begin to see positive movement and recognition in your professional life, you will grow less complacent at work.
- If you are in your own business, step up your game, redefine your goals, and take things to the next level. Reinvent yourself. If necessary, begin reinventing your company.
- If you are retired and are bored out of your mind, commit to a new project, get involved somewhere that you have passion, and engage in life again.
- If you have grown complacent in your personal life, consider taking up a new sport or hobby. What have you always wanted to do? Rediscover an old passion. Maybe you liked to go boating as a kid. How about skiing, karate or playing cards? Connect with your surroundings. Change things up and take on any type of new activity that is invigorating to you. Choose something that brings your passion back.

In summary, you break through complacency patterns by setting new goals for yourself and following through on them. You are invigorated by a variety of new commitments and experiences that stimulate your spirit and by generating results that show you are still effective in the world. You discover that you can still explore new horizons, whether they are personal or professional. When my children were young, I was unable to go snow skiing as often as I liked. Living in Atlanta, far from the mountains, it seemed like too much of a burden to make an exciting ski trip happen. As my kids grew up, I made the commitment and took the initiative to take everyone on an incredible family ski vacation at least once a year. Everyone got into it and now we all look forward to going. Over the years, we have taken some amazing ski vacations together. It is something we look forward to enjoying together for the rest of our lives. Now I am not complacent about my Play Time anymore. The passion is back and at a higher level than ever.

You will know you are escaping a complacency pattern when you start to feel like a kid again—a kid with a new toy. You are excited and passionate about your extended life.

DEP #4: COMFORT PATTERNS

Life is good. You've worked hard, and you are successful—both professionally and personally. You respect yourself and are surrounded by good people. You've got good habits and a routine that works. But, could it be that your level of comfort is also creating some dis-ease? Deep down, do you think there is more that you would love to experience? Is the comfort beginning to hurt?

When you are in a comfort pattern, you are all about maintaining the status quo. You revel in past successes. Unlike the fiery perseverance that got you to where you are today, now you want to avoid making waves. You are generally no longer striving. You feel your days of hard work are behind you—but so is the pleasure of challenging yourself and being in the game. The tire around your waste and hips is starting to expand as your comfort throws you out of balance.

The challenge of a comfort pattern is that it is easy to go from being on a roll to getting in a rut. You generally stop living up to your potential and it is easy to lose your edge.

Living The 100 Year Lifestyle
Weight Loss and The 100 Year Lifestyle

I know about these patterns because, to some degree, I have lived them all–as we all have. In my own life, when I grew comfortable, I also grew fat. I gained close to 40 pounds. I remember preparing a video for my son's thirteenth birthday and looking at myself on the video thinking, *Who is that whale wearing my bathing suit?* My first thought was to lose weight. But there was something about the thought of having a primary goal of *losing* that did not work for me. I had never wanted to "lose" anything, or "lose" at anything before in my life. I never wanted to lose a game of sports, I never wanted to lose anything valuable, and I never wanted to lose in business. I always wanted to win.

I was always one of those people motivated by quality of life. I decided that while the extra weight was going to come off my body, it wasn't mine to begin with. It was just an extra burden that I was carrying around that it was time to unload. I decided to develop a new relationship with my abdomen and say goodbye to the extra burden while welcoming all the exciting things that I was going to gain by my commitment to my own human potential pattern. I started saying no to all the foods that tasted good for 30 seconds but were bad for me. I got my "edge" by calling them liars when they would talk to me and tell me to eat them. I started making food and exercise choices that supported my ideal 100 Year lifestyle. I started focusing on all the things I was gaining, including more energy, feeling younger, being more active, sleeping better, breathing better, looking younger and healthier, and feeling like a kid again. My desire for quality of life kept the feelings of being deprived away that many people who are trying to lose weight often experience. Occasionally I got off track and then got back on track with my next choice (Life Changing Principle #2), knowing that the desire for quality of life gives me lasting motivation and a sense of winning that is greater than the 30 seconds of sweetness that might be provided from a sugar addiction. Ten years later, I have kept the extra 40 pounds from finding their way back to my body and am practicing and living my ideal 100 Year Lifestyle. I know what you may be going through. If I can do it, you can too.

You often come across people like this in a professional capacity. One example is the doctor who has a good reputation in the community, but suddenly he or she stops investing in the latest techniques and technologies to educate and help patients. You also see this with politicians who strive to get into office by focusing on the needs of the people, and then lose their connection with their constituency. Indeed, when most people look back on their lives, the best times often happen during their "up and coming" years. Too much comfort can really set your life out of balance. Keep that edge. Always look for new ways to make a contribution and use your talents to make a difference. The 100 Year Lifestyle is about achieving the ultimate balance and enjoying that balance for a lifetime.

One character I have always loved is Pigpen from the Peanuts cartoons. Pigpen has a cloud of dirt that surrounds him wherever he goes. When he is moving, the cloud lags behind him. When he stops moving the cloud of dust catches up to him and gets in his mouth, eyes, and nose. If you are used to being an achiever and you slow down, be on the lookout for the clouds of negativity, boredom, and pessimism that can often come from settling into a comfort pattern. This is often the case when someone retires.

The challenge and opportunity of comfort is to reconnect with a sense of purpose that inspires you while balancing yourself with the Play Time you want. Be careful not to let the comfort become so comfortable that it leads to complacency. When you get stuck in this pattern, you can lose your creativity, sabotage your relationships, or become negative.

Centenarian Secret

You will be truly happy and passionate when you are fully engaged in your life again. Not as a robot, doing things the way you always have in the past, but by embracing your life consciously based on what you know you love to do, your worldliness, and experience. Start thinking "outside the box" again for this next phase of your life.

Build spontaneity into your life by the way you choose to spend your time, the places you go, and the people with whom you choose to spend your time. Pursue the projects, innovation, travel, and time with your family and friends that you have been dreaming about. Get out of your comfort zone and don't let the dust settle unless it is on your terms. Your 100 Year Lifestyle is just waiting for you to fan its flames. Use your talents and learn new skills. Enjoy and explore the global playground that is about to be yours as a result of your commitment to your 100 Year Lifestyle.

DEP #5: THE HUMAN POTENTIAL PATTERN: THE SECRET TO A SENSATIONAL CENTURY

In this pattern, you're energized about your life. You've got good health, habits, and relationships. You're giving as much or more than you are receiving. You invite change. Your actions are aligned with your life's purpose. You have a done the work to establish a pattern of thoughts and actions that consciously support your highest values and Innate potential.

One of the things that attracted me to a career in chiropractic when I was younger was the sense of purpose that I saw in the doctors I met. Chiropractors seemed to be inspired to express their own Innate potential, while also providing the care for their patients to help them do the same. This was very different from the very Crisis Care only approach that I saw in the medical status quo. When I went to Life Chiropractic College, now Life University, and studied chiropractic philosophy, I understood why. I discovered that optimizing the expression of your Innate Intelligence and human potential is built into the foundation of the principles and the care. It became very exciting for me to see the patients and doctors that I work with realize that potential, and it is exciting to know that you will have the opportunity to experience this too.

How do you make your human potential pattern a habit? It begins with your first thought of the day, first action, first feeling. You will find that your day goes much better when you consciously start out in this pattern. Here's a sample scenario where every choice is conscious and builds on the next.

> **First Thought:** It's good to be alive. I am healing today. I have energy. I am manifesting abundance in my life through my work and my relationships.
>
> **First Action:** Stretch, feel your entire body, breathe deeply, pray, and connect to your goals.
>
> **First Feeling:** Experience gratitude, excitement, passion, and hope.

Your energy will dramatically increase when you make your human potential pattern your lifestyle. You will become so energized that even your Play Time will be filled with more energy. You will need less sleep, less food, and enjoy more of what life has to offer.

DIRECTING YOUR NEW-FOUND ENERGY INTO YOUR 100 YEAR LIFESTYLE

You have an opportunity to redistribute your energy now because you want to, not because your life depends on it. Your old dominant energy patterns can be consciously broken.

Who you will become in the next phase of your life is a direct reflection of how you choose to distribute your energy. You can begin by monitoring your energy and your attitude and shifting toward your human potential.

HAVE A 100 PERCENT CONSCIOUS DAY

Try this today. From the time you wake up in the morning, until the time you go to bed at night, be aware of every moment. Become fully aware of your environment, your emotions, and your activities. You may find that some of who you are and what you do is unconscious, out of control, and not what you would choose for the rest of your life. Some of these things can be changed immediately. If you find yourself trying to control others, or being controlled by others, stop it. Learn to approach your relationships from a place of acceptance, love, and kindness. Make it a policy to only pursue relationships with people who share those same values. Have the same attitude about other behaviors like eating and drinking. If you eat or drink unconsciously, stop before this becomes an addiction. Food and drink are among the great pleasures of life. You deserve to enjoy them, as you would any other relationship—from a place of appreciation, respect, and balance.

INCREASE ENERGY AWARENESS USING YOUR BREATHING

One way to increase your awareness of your dominant energy pattern is to monitor your breathing, which is a great indicator of how you are consciously or unconsciously directing your energy. To do this, take a deep breath and feel the full range of motion with your lungs. Go ahead and take another deep breath right now. When we get overwhelmed, our breathing gets shallow and our chest can get tight and rigid around our lungs. Tune into your breathing throughout the day. See if you can catch yourself when you are taking shallow breaths and immediately take some deep ones. Paying attention to the full range of motion in your lungs can immediately bring you to a state of awareness, stop a destructive pattern in its tracks, and give you an opportunity to choose a new pattern.

INCREASE ENERGY AWARENESS USING YOUR HEART RATE

Monitoring your heart rate is also a great way to become conscious of your dominant energy patterns and how they are affecting your body. Wear a heart monitor, and as you go throughout your day, check your heart rate every 30 minutes. Take note of what causes your heart rate to go up and down. When you feel your intensity rising, look at your heart rate. See if it's rising. If it is, take a deep breath and let the tension out of your body. You will see your heart rate drop back down again. This is a great way to become aware of your unconscious patterns and how they affect you, and immediately gain control over them. When people survive a heart attack, the crisis motivates them to exercise with a heart monitor. Why not do this now as a way to improve your quality of life?

INCREASE ENERGY AWARENESS USING POSTURE

Your posture is another great way to catch yourself in a pattern that is less than ideal. Do you ever find yourself slouching at your computer, while you are talking on the phone, watching television, or eating a meal? When I mention posture in my seminars it is amazing how instantaneously everyone all of a sudden straightens up. You should tune into your posture regularly throughout the day and when you catch yourself slouching, shift your posture immediately. Train yourself to sit and stand erect. This opens your lungs, is good for your spine, and makes you more confident. Chronic slouching or discomfort when you are erect is one of the signs that your spine may be unbalanced with interference to the function of your nervous system, a condition known as Vertebral Subluxation. Remember, in the world of The 100 Year Lifestyle, when you are out of balance, you are broke. If you have this condition now, it will only get worse over time and can severely affect your health and quality of life now and as you age. I see this in my practice all the time and this can be corrected with chiropractic care.

CHANGE YOUR PATTERN, CHANGE YOUR LIFE

Like the clothes in your wardrobe, you may wear one energy pattern 20 percent of the time and another 80 percent. Notice what pattern you are in most of the time. Does it suit your current goals? Is it moving you quickly or slowly toward them? Is there another route you would rather take? If so, then change course. Change your posture, breathing, and relax your heart. Take a different action. Choose your new human potential pattern with your ideal 100 Year Lifestyle in mind.

STAY HIGH

Here are some additional tips to help you switch into and sustain high energy to fuel your 100 Year Lifestyle. I'm not talking about hyperactive energy. What I'm talking about is a focused, calm, naturally high state of energy that comes from an inner awareness of your own human potential. You can power your 100 Year Lifestyle:

BY EATING HIGH-ENERGY FOODS:
- Whole grains
- Fresh fruits and vegetables
- Lean meats, fish, and poultry
- Vegetable proteins

- Miso, edamame, flaxseed oil
- Vitamin and mineral supplements

BY ENGAGING IN HIGH-ENERGY ACTIVITIES:

- Fun exercise
- Getting six to eight hours of restful sleep each night
- Meaningful work
- Quality time with family and friends
- Volunteerism and community service
- Yoga, Martial Arts, and Pilates
- Chiropractic adjustments for Lifestyle Care
- Getting a new pet
- Change-of-pace activities like holding a staff meeting outside, going on a walk with neighbors, taking up a new sport like skiing, cycling, swimming, or boating

BY MAINTAINING HIGH-ENERGY THOUGHTS, AFFIRMATIONS AND ATTITUDES:

- I am happy
- I am healthy
- I am motivated
- I am passionate
- I am grateful
- I am focused
- I am faithful
- I am worthy

Of course, it's not enough to choose high-energy food, activities, and thoughts. You must also avoid energy drainers such as:

EATING LOW-ENERGY FOODS:

- Processed foods
- Fast foods
- Junk foods
- Sugary desserts
- Foods made with white flour or sugar
- Fried foods

ENGAGING IN LOW-ENERGY ACTIVITIES:

- Channel surfing or mindless Web surfing
- Difficult, dull, or stressful work
- Investing time in meaningless relationships
- Wasteful spending
- Falling into a boring routine and losing touch with the fun of life
- Arguing unnecessarily

GETTING CAUGHT UP ON LOW-ENERGY THOUGHTS AND ACTIONS:

- I don't accept my current situation and circumstances.
- I don't have faith.
- I don't have what it takes to reach my goals.
- I can't make a fresh start every day.
- I can't choose my pattern at any time.
- I can't get off track and get back on track with my next choice.
- I am not learning every day.
- I am not grateful for all my experiences.
- My challenges don't teach me the lessons I need to learn.
- Why bother?
- I am a victim.

IMAGINE THE POSSIBILITY

You've done an amazing job of opening your mind to the possibilities of change. By committing to a sensational century or more of life, you are choosing to express your Innate Intelligence to its full potential. You are deciding what you want to experience, what condition you want to be in, and what will top your list of achievements along the way. Living a 100 Year Lifestyle will optimize your health, life, love, and relationships as you establish a powerful legacy to live long and strong.

As you find the energy to change, don't worry if things aren't different overnight. Just stay true to the journey, know that you will get there and your new high-energy human potential pattern will drive the process to your ideal 100 Year Lifestyle.

DISCOVER YOUR POTENTIAL
ACTION PLAN FOR LASTING CHANGE

1. Take your Personal Energy Inventory and become aware of all of the places that you let your energy leak out into the atmosphere. Choose energy-enhancing thoughts, actions, and feelings and begin to make them a part of who you are.

2. Decide which Dominant Energy Pattern you are in and begin to identify your personal human potential pattern. Begin making choices following the Three Life-Changing Principles that support your ideal 100 Year Lifestyle where you are living at your best every day.

3. Make The Midstream Catch a habit. Have a 100 percent conscious day. Take it all in and be honest with yourself about when you are destructive, in survival, complacent, comfortable, and when you are at your best. Begin to let go of the things about you that are destructive and rewire yourself for the rest of your 100 years.

4. Choose energy-enhancing first thoughts, actions, and feelings and reinforce them throughout the day with personal affirmations.

5. Monitor your breathing, heart rate, and posture. Begin with your breathing and posture immediately because they do not require any equipment. When you are ready, invest in a heart monitor and tune into your heart rate. You will be amazed what you learn about yourself during this process.

6. Choose high-energy foods and activities. When given the choice of low-energy foods and activities, choose high energy. Choose a power walk over being a couch potato. Choose high-energy foods over low-energy foods. Choose healthy interactions with other people rather than destructive interactions.

7. Stop and choose. When you catch yourself unconsciously doing things that you know you want to change, shift your energy. Literally say to yourself *stop* and physically and emotionally stop yourself. Now make a new choice that supports your ideal 100 Year Lifestyle. Initially you may feel like a tennis ball bouncing back and forth 100 times a day. Eventually you will settle into your human potential pattern, and it will be your lifestyle. You will love it.

PART 3

The Commonsense Strategy of The 100 Year Lifestyle!

We all have a history. I don't want yours and you don't want mine. What's more important than your history is your commitment.

CHAPTER 5

STOP KILLING YOURSELF!

If you want to live an active, healthy, quality life for 80, 90, 100 years and beyond, there is absolutely, positively one thing you are going to have to do. Do you know what that one thing is? Are you ready for this one? This is profound, yet simple—both at the same time. You are going to have to not die. So . . .

Stop Killing Yourself!

There are so many ways that we kill ourselves both quickly and slowly, every day, taking years off our lives and life out of our years. We do this through the small and seemingly insignificant decisions that we make that enhance or detract from our quality of life. We eat the extra cookie, even though we might not even taste it. We skip our evening workout because we are tired, even though we know the workout will energize us. We slump over keyboards all day without moving around and stretching out our legs. We develop habits and ignore the minor problems until they become a crisis. What's wrong with this? The problem is that many of us do these things every day—often with the intention of turning over a new leaf. But it's not the resolutions that matter; it's the actions we take every day. It's those very destructive actions or inactions, done over time, that are literally killing us slowly over time. Understand that we have the potential to live a quality 100 years. But many of us will never realize this potential and even worse, run the risk of rotting away for a decade or more in a nursing home if we don't take better care of ourselves.

Centenarian Secret
There are now around 450 people living who are 110-plus years of age. The most super-centenarians are in the United States, United Kingdom, Japan, France and Italy. None of these people planned to live this long. They just never died.

I hear people say, "I don't want to live to 100". Well first of all, you may not have a choice. Secondly, this is not a good excuse for being self-destructive and not taking responsibility for your health and your choices. If not 100, what is your number that you want to die? Is it 74, 86, 93, 108? If you were healthy and enjoying your life, why would you want to go? You wouldn't. Remember, the number 100 is a representation of possibility and your Innate potential which in your case could be even higher. Your M-PYR, minimum potential years remaining, is not your maximum. Based on your family history, we know the *minimum* is possible for you and you might live even longer.

The real issue that The 100 Year Lifestyle tackles is not actually when we die or what we die from, but how we live and the choices that we make while we are living. It's about quality of life every day! We've all heard a story of a woman, or man, who exercised regularly, ate the right foods, and then goes out for a jog one day and drops dead of a heart attack. While this is certainly sad and shocking, it is also rare. Jogging is not one of the leading causes of death in this country or any other country. This is not a good excuse to continue down a path of self-destruction. Many of us justify our poor choices, day in and day out, with stories like this one. We use them as justification for destructive patterns of self-abuse and we use them to build a case against ourselves for why we don't change.

One of my patients was a money manager for a large investment-banking firm. He would come to my chiropractic office for adjustments when he was in a crisis. He had several areas of vertebral subluxation, spinal injuries with nerve interference, and they were causing his back pain, nerve problems and deterioration to progress over the years. He was completely out of shape and nearly every organ in his body was unhealthy and not functioning properly. He struggled getting his extra 40 pounds on and off the adjusting table. He came to see me two to three times per year because the adjustments were able to put out his fires. We were able to calm the crisis. Lifestyle Care was not even in his consciousness even though his family was healthy, fully engaged in their Lifestyle Care, had been getting adjusted for years, and were enjoying the benefits of living The 100 Year Lifestyle. Preventative health care was like a foreign language to him. Unfortunately, no matter how hard I tried to convince him that he was headed for more serious trouble if he didn't make the Critical Transition to Lifestyle Care, he wouldn't listen. When I asked him why he wasn't willing to be more proactive about his health, he told me the story about the jogger. What a ridiculous excuse to perpetuate his suffering. He would only make his health a priority when his suffering—crisis motivation—kicked in at its highest level.

Living The 100 Year Lifestyle is not simply about not dying; it is about the quality of your life every day. Nobody I have ever met has driven by a nursing home and said, "That's where I'd like to end up." We don't just "end up" in there; we kill ourselves slowly over time. This man was suffering on so many levels because of his lack of commitment to his own health and wellbeing. He would say things like, "I want to just live for today" and "I just want to enjoy my life." But what's enjoyable about feeling like you're going to pass out every time you walk up a flight of stairs? What's enjoyable about working yourself into the ground without enjoying good times with your family and friends along the way? Every choice you make to produce a quality 100 Year Lifestyle will also improve the quality of your life today.

A Choice That Changed a Teenager's Life
Submitted by Brandon Roberts, D.C.

Emily, a 16 year old student, was in crisis. She had suffered through life with severe allergies and asthma and was on about a dozen medications to treat these conditions. The newest prescription was for a corticosteroid which had caused her to gain about 20 pounds. The symptoms were not going away even with all the medications and she was scheduled to have her tonsils and adenoids removed then have her sinuses scraped soon after. Emily was done living the 40 to 50 year lifestyle which is living from one crisis to another to yet another. She was ready to make the Critical Transition to The 100 Year Lifestyle.

Within a week of her first chiropractic exam and adjustment, Emily noticed that she needed her inhaler less frequently. Within a month, she was breathing more easily, her sense of smell was better and she was down to using only a couple of the medications. She could not recall the last time she needed to reach for her inhaler. After two months and staying consistent with her chiropractic check-ups, she was off all her medications and was able to cancel the surgeries.

Emily continues her Lifestyle Care and is excited about living her ideal 100 Year Lifestyle. She has been able to completely discontinue using allergy and asthma medications and has not required surgery. Can you imagine what her life would have been like otherwise?

I was recently flying back from Philadelphia after giving a keynote speech to a group of doctors, and I sat next to a musician who was coming back from a gig. We talked about his music career and his family for a while. He was about 100 pounds overweight and not taking care of his body at all. His diet consisted completely of junk food. He told me that he ate too much and drank too much. As our discussion progressed he asked me what I did for a living. I told him that I was a chiropractor, author and a professional speaker. I told him about this book. He told me that he knew that he needed to make changes in his life, and he already knew what they were. He said his unhealthy lifestyle was causing tremendous suffering. He had shortness of breath, back and neck pain, fatigue, and excessive stress—not to mention the strain on his heart, spine and nervous system was too much to bear.

He then told me about his 98-year-old grandfather, who was still in good health and enjoying life. He realized he had the same genetic potential as his grandfather, but he also knew that he had to take responsibility and *stop killing himself* today, or he wasn't going to come close to fulfilling his longevity potential. His M-PYR scared the crap out of him. Shortly before we departed, he told me that he was going to start making some "serious changes now." Otherwise, he said, he wasn't going to make it. He was scared of the potential pain and suffering that lie ahead and he really wanted to start living life to the fullest. I told him I wished him well. He had an exciting road ahead. The resolution he made that day was easy. All the little choices he would make from that day forward would determine his success or failure down the road. Three months later I called to see how he was doing and he was thrilled. He told me that he had begun to make the changes that would get him back on track. He had lost 15 pounds, replaced the post-gig midnight eating and drinking binges with a power walk, he stopped popping over-the-counter pain pills and he had started seeing a chiropractor to get his spine and nervous system healthy. He was excited about the possibility of living 100 healthy years. He said to me passionately, "I've got a lot of music in me."

LIVE LONG AND STRONG
Stop Killing Yourself.
Effective immediately, I will stop killing myself by eliminating the following habits that I know are not good for me.

_____

_____

_____

_____

You, too, have a lot of music in you. In the next few pages we'll take a look at the leading causes of death in this country. You will see that these are not the leading cause of death in all countries. You will also see that the majority of these conditions are preventable if you are willing to live The 100 Year Lifestyle. As you look at the list you may find yourself making a comment like "that's what my father died from." You may even say, "My grandparents died from that," and "This disease runs in my family."

Even though our parents and grandparents may have passed away from diseases with a genetic component to them, your parents probably outlived your grandparents by a good 5, 10, 20, or even 30 years. The important thing to remember is, for most of us, we not only inherited a set of genes, but we inherited a way of thinking and living as well—a lifestyle. In our generation, for example, we see a lot of stressed-out parents—"hyper-parents"—struggling to balance work and kids. Times have changed, but instead of connecting with and realigning our values, we just paddle harder. Our unwillingness to change with changing times keeps us in survival and destructive energy patterns that take years off of our life, and life from our years.

Think of someone trying to dance to disco even after the music has changed to rap. You would see a whirlwind of activity, in all the wrong directions. This is what happens when we resist change—the toll it takes on our minds, bodies, and spirits can be very damaging. This leads to a 60, 70 or 80 Year Lifestyle versus The 100 Year Lifestyle.

The average life expectancy for men in the US, currently, is just 75 years for men and 82 for women. In Monaco, the country with the highest life expectancy in the world, it is 85 for men and 93 for women. Australia's numbers are 79 and 84 and the UK's are 78 and 82 respectively. The ranking for the U.S. is now 51st versus its ranking of 42nd in 2007 when the first edition of The 100 Year Lifestyle came out. You can get the Life Expectancy for all countries at the CIA World Factbook online.

Life Expectancy Ranking by Country
#1   Monaco
#3   Japan
#9   Australia
#12 Canada
#15 Spain
#18 Israel
#19 Iceland
#25 New Zealand
#29 Jordan
#30 United Kingdom
#41 South Korea
#44 Puerto Rico
#45 Bosnia
#50 Guam
#51 United States
https://www.cia.gov/library/publications/the-world-factbook/rankorder/2102rank.html

"Average" means that some people are living much longer, and some people are dying much younger. Where will your life expectancy fall and even more importantly, what will your quality of life be along the way? The health choices you make today will absolutely impact your quality of life now and in the future?

You are designed to thrive as you age and you will if you listen to your body's Innate Intelligence, trust yourself, start making healthier choices and make the changes you know you need to make. After all, life is a series of transitions, and the one you are about to go on—embracing the reality of your potential longevity—can be the most exciting time of your life. Confront the unknown with the knowledge that on the other side of change is a tremendous feeling of freedom, youthfulness, and renewal. This is where you will thrive. Remember Life Changing Principle# 1: Change is easy. Thinking about change is hard.

Centenarian Secret
Only around half of centenarians have had first-degree relatives or grandparents who also achieved very old age. Many have exceptionally old siblings.

LISTEN TO YOUR BODY'S INNATE INTELLIGENCE

Your mind, body, and spirit are amazing. They are driven to thrive by an Innate Intelligence, an inner wisdom that makes approximately 8,000,000 new blood cells in your bone marrow every second. Your bones are constantly rebuilding themselves and are not at all static. Your heart beats an average of 60 times per minute, or an incredible 3 billion times over the course of 100 years. We now know that your brain cells can renew and develop new pathways even into adulthood. Studies have shown that to build your incredible body from scratch would drain all the treasures of the world with no guarantee of success. Why would you kill yourself slowly over time and deteriorate your original parts. It's time to stop killing yourself and start keeping yourself functioning at your highest level. In my chiropractic practice, I've made a career of watching people embrace this philosophy and fall in love with their results. You will too.

Your Innate wisdom is trying to assert itself every day, trying to guide you to what is best for you. Did your parents and grandparents test the limits of their genetic potential? Probably not even close. Your M-PYR, Minimum Potential Years Remaining, is not your Max-PYR. It is not your maximum. Do not use your family history as a reason to not live The 100 Year Lifestyle you deserve.

Instead, let's look at choices that support your longevity and maximize your quality of life every day. I understand that you may make sacrifices on occasion for the sake of your family or work. Sacrifices are inevitable. But make them from a place of awareness and get back on track with your next choice.

As a society, we are very focused on the external. We spend our days striving to achieve external worth, while slowly killing ourselves on the inside. This is a destructive pattern. The decisions that have the greatest impact on your health are not the big ones, like starting a new diet. They are the seemingly insignificant ones you make day to day that perpetuate destructive patterns and kill you slowly over time.

Your genes play a role in your longevity, but a much smaller one than you would think—they comprise less than a third of the variables leading to longevity. If you explore the top killers of people in our society today, you'll find that most are preventable through healthy lifestyle choices that are good for you. People have a greater chance of living to be 100 when they stay relatively healthy throughout their lives. As the New England Centenarian Study learned in their research, 90 percent of centenarians have been functionally independent the vast majority of their lives, up until the average age of 92 years.

> **Centenarian Secret**
> "Centenarians disprove the perception that 'the older you get, the sicker you get,' centenarians teach us that the older you get the healthier you've been."–The New England Centenarian Study.

A smaller percentage of centenarians make it after overcoming a serious illness. But they are the exception and not the rule. For most of these people, crisis motivated them to change. But why not avoid the crisis to begin with? Why put yourself in a position to need a modern-day miracle. There are very few magic bullets. The way you care for yourself, and the environment in which you live, will have the greatest impact on your health and longevity. Patients and colleagues used to tell me all the time after getting a series of adjustments, "You are a miracle worker, Doc." The truth is that the miracle is actually within you. It is your Innate Intelligence that has the power to heal you and get you functioning at the highest levels of health and vitality, as long as it is not interfered with. As a chiropractor, I always felt honored to work with this healing power within each person and help people optimize it throughout their lifetime. Wouldn't it be great to nurture this intelligence to keep yourself healthy each day? You bet it would!

Centenarian Secret

Many centenarian women have had children after the age of 35 and even 40 years of age. Having children after 40 may be a sign that a woman's reproductive system is aging slowly—and that the rest of her body is aging slowly as well. Additionally, women who have children after 40 have four times a greater chance of living to 100.

You will be excited to learn that the leading causes of death are all preventable. While you may have some of them in your family history, the commonsense and proven strategies that follow may help you to postpone them for decades or even wipe them out of your future completely.

CHAPTER 6

AVOIDING THE TOP TEN LEADING CAUSES OF PREVENTABLE DEATH

We all know that people die every day. According to the U.S. National Center for Health Statistics, 2,436,682 people died in the year 2009. Of these, 1,217,047 of them were men and 1,219,635 of them were female. The leading causes of death were heart disease, cancer, cerebrovascular diseases like stroke, chronic lower respiratory diseases, Alzheimer's, diabetes, the flu, and pneumonia. If you are like many people, you probably have at least a little concern about one of these conditions. For example, your father may have died of a heart attack, and now you fear dying from one as well. Maybe your mother or grandparents suffered from cancer and the thought of you experiencing the same fate is a little scary. Their destiny does not have to be yours.

It's important to understand that disease generally does not jump out of the closet at you. If you are paying attention to your Innate Intelligence, you will be alerted when something is amiss. Typically, you experience some sort of physical or mental disharmony or "dis-ease" before you get sick. Maybe you feel out of balance and fatigue sets in. Your digestion or elimination patterns may change. When you heed the early warning signs, and take the steps to get your body functioning at its highest level through proactive health care and lifestyle strategies, you can often prevent them from occurring in the first place. It makes much more sense to optimize your body's natural defense system. Too often, we shift into self-care only after we experience symptoms of disease. This is not very effective, as symptoms are often the last sign of a serious problem. This is crisis motivation. In a state of homeostasis, the body fights off disease and infection on its own. It keeps your arteries clean and it eliminates rabid cells that can turn into cancer. Work with your body's natural ability to function properly, keep it in balance, and enjoy a 100 health years. In fact, many of The 100 Year Lifestyle Affiliate chiropractors teach this program in their communities as a service. Inquire when this is happening in your area and attend with your family and friends.

In the following section, we will take a look at the leading causes of death in this country. Again, what's interesting is that these are not the leading causes of death in all countries. We are going to talk about some of the lifestyle and health care differences in nations around the world and how you might be able to incorporate some of these changes into your own life, today, as part of your 100 Year Lifestyle.

Do you realize the degree of control you have over your health? If you have a genetic disposition to any type of life-threatening condition, fearlessly take the proactive steps to reduce the chance that it will affect your life and live your life to the fullest. This commonsense strategy is exciting and I encourage you to passionately pursue knowledge like this throughout your life. Making lifestyle changes can be a healthier option than taking a handful of drugs every day.

Centenarian Secret
Pomegranate juice may help reduce cholesterol. Turmeric may help prevent Alzheimer's.

MANAGING YOUR HEALTH TO 100 YEARS AND BEYOND

Let's take a look at preventative measures you can take against the leading causes of death. This information has been condensed here for your easy access and implementation. The solutions that are presented are not a mystery that was just discovered. They are well documented scientifically and are just waiting for you to make them a part of your lifestyle.

HEART DISEASE

According to the National Health and Nutrition Examination Survey, 76 million adults have high blood pressure, and an astounding 98 million have high cholesterol. Heart disease is the leading cause of death for men and women in this country. Men tend to develop it at high percentages sooner than women. This is why it's traditionally considered more of a "male" problem—many men die from it in their prime.

Comparatively, heart disease is not the leading cause of death in places like Okinawa, Japan. Okinawans have 80 percent fewer heart attacks than North Americans. When they have a heart attack, they are twice as likely to survive. However, when they migrate to this country and adopt our lifestyle, they take on our same arterial risk. How much more do you need to know? Take heart. It's largely about choices. Even if you have currently been diagnosed with heart disease, it has been shown that you can help reverse it through good nutrition and 100 Year Lifestyle choices.

There are some obvious ways to prevent heart disease. First, we know that you can reduce your risk of heart disease by not smoking. Maintaining a healthy weight is also key. Pear-shaped figures have less heart disease than "apple-shaped" figures, which are so common among middle-aged men. A diet rich in fruits and vegetables and low in fat is very important. There are tricks you will discover as you learn more about diet. For example, pomegranate juice can, in fact, help reduce your cholesterol, and three grams of Omega-3 fatty acids a day are good for the heart. I encourage you to read everything you can about heart-healthy fitness and nutrition and reduce your stress levels. Living a heart-healthy lifestyle will support you in achieving your 100 Year Lifestyle.

Seriously consider exercise, nutrition, and other forms of holistic approaches to change your lifestyle prior to taking medication. If your doctor does suggest you start a heart medication regimen, always learn about the potential long term side effects. Get a second opinion. Also, look for lifestyle changes that you can make to avoid them completely. Speak to your doctor if you have a family history of heart disease, and develop a plan that will serve your goals for your extended life. If you depend on medication without changing your lifestyle, you will probably be stuck in that regimen for the next 30, 40, or 50 years and the side effects can be scary.

Here are some other basic guidelines:

- Don't smoke or use other tobacco products.
- Eat a varied diet, rich in fruits, vegetables, and low-fat foods.
- Maintain a healthy weight.
- Consume alcohol in moderation.
- Get at least 30 minutes of aerobic exercise three to five days per week.
- Keep your blood chemistry levels in normal ranges.
- Control your blood sugar if you have diabetes.
- Control your blood chemistry levels with diet and exercise before committing to a lifetime of medication.
- Relax. Eliminate physical and emotional stressors.

- Monitor your blood chemistry, heart rate, and blood pressure.
- Keep your spine and nervous system healthy and functioning without interference
- Implement the Health Care Hierarchy of The 100 Year Lifestyle in the next chapter.

CANCER

Cancer is the second leading cause of death for men and women. Lung cancer is the most common type of cancer. Approximately 200,000 Americans are diagnosed each year. Around 87 percent of lung cancer is linked to cigarette smoking. Prostate cancer is also very common. Scientists believe that hereditary prostate cancer accounts for just 9 percent of all cases. A high-fat diet is believed to be a contributing factor. Prostate cancer is very rare in places like Okinawa, where the diet tends to be low in fat.

Breast cancer rates are also very rare there, as they are throughout most of Japan. Scientists think that a key factor is the daily consumption of phytoestrogens through natural sources like miso. In fact, many men with prostate cancer in the United States now make phytoestrogen-rich flaxseed and flaxseed oil a part of their diets. Tomatoes—a rich source of lycopene—also mitigate chances of prostate cancer. I encourage you to read everything you can about nutrition and lifestyle to prevent cancer and keep your body functioning at its highest level. Don't stop with the news. Lifelong learning is a key component of The 100 Year Lifestyle.

Here are some basic guidelines:
- Don't smoke or use other tobacco products.
- Eat a varied diet, rich in fruits, vegetables, fiber, and low-fat foods. Don't just eat healthy foods out of the fear of getting sick. Eat to enjoy and promote a healthy 100 Year Lifestyle.
- Avoid Genetically Modified Foods (GMOs)

- Maintain a healthy weight.
- Get at least 30 minutes of exercise three to five days per week.
- Avoid overexposure to the sun.
- Drink alcohol only in moderation.
- Be aware of potential cancer-causing substances (carcinogens) in your home and workplace, and take steps to reduce your exposure to these substances. Common household cleaning products and cosmetics may contain ingredients known to cause cancer. Take the time to do some research.
- Know your family health history and have regular preventive health screenings in the areas related to your history.
- Keep your spine and nervous system healthy and functioning without interference.
- Implement the Health Care Hierarchy of The 100 Year Lifestyle in the next chapter.

Are you beginning to see that most of these items qualify as common sense? Avoiding these healthy choices causes dis-ease, disharmony, weakness, and imbalance that stresses your nervous system and heart, and makes you less adaptable to the world around you. Your energy is redistributed and goes toward survival and battling the negative impact of the dis-ease rather than on optimizing your Innate Intelligence. Your body's capabilities get redirected and diverted.

ACCIDENTS

Talk about preventable! Accidents are a leading cause of death in this country. In fact, accidents rank third among the leading causes of death for men. Certainly there are many unavoidable dangers in the world. Things happen. But you have to look no further than a mountain biking trail to see how many men are wired. We love to test our limits, and then some. Although car accidents remain the most pervasive risk for accidental deaths, men are almost twice as likely as women to drive drunk—another avoidable risk. To reduce your chances of a fatal crash:

- Wear your seat belt.
- Keep your speed down.
- Practice defensive driving.
- Don't drive while sleepy or under the influence of drugs or alcohol, this includes prescription drugs.

Poisoning is the second leading cause of fatal accidents to men. To reduce your risk of poisoning:

- Place carbon monoxide and smoke detectors near bedrooms in your house.
- Have fuel-burning appliances inspected each year.
- Store household products in their original containers.
- Read and follow label instructions for household products.
- Stop the pill popping. Stop the destructive pattern of popping a pill every time you feel a symptom. Let your body heal itself. If you absolutely have to take medication, make sure you follow label instructions carefully and practice self-care and health care strategies to minimize their need and offset potential side effects.
- Ventilate areas where you use chemical products.

Post the poison control number, (800) 222-1222, by each telephone in your home, especially if you have children or grandchildren.

The Dangers of Prescriptions Drugs

Choosing to mask symptoms creates an additional risk to your health through side effects. Before you pop another pill, you must understand how medication side effects *directly* affect your body today and in years to come.

Medications are tested in a laboratory until the chemical reaction that they are designed to achieve is reproducible. The direct effects of this lab testing must be consistent before these chemicals are ever tested on animals or people. Once human testing begins, scientists measure the impact of these medications to see if they cause the same direct effects that were induced in a laboratory. If these effects are reproducible, the testing continues to see if any other effects occur.

These are called 'side effects' because they were not present in the laboratory setting and their impact on humans was outside of their intended effect. In actuality, these side effects are direct effects of these drugs on the body. Because we are all unique in our body chemistry, direct effects, labeled side effects, impact people differently, and they are much more common than people think.

Drug companies prepare a list of side effects for the consumer, while also listing additional side effects that doctors should be aware of. If you go to www.drugs.com and type in any drug, then select "Side Effects" you will notice that the side effects/direct effects for the physician to be aware of might be up to a dozen pages. Most people are unaware of all the effects that medications can cause, and often treat these symptoms with other drugs. this is dangerous because the interactions between drugs can cause even more severe direct effects. Too many people unknowingly go down this road until their body chemistry and health is completely screwed up.

The direct effects of these medications, combined with the reality of our extended life spans of 80, 90, 100 years and beyond, makes it obvious that living a lifestyle that keeps you independently healthy and free from the need for medications is your best long-term option.

Do a side effect/direct effect check right now on www.drugs.com and seriously consider a drug-free alternative.

Falls and drowning are also leading causes of fatal injury. Commonsense precautions include using a safety ladder, placing nonskid mats in showers and tubs, and never swimming alone. Also, many fatal injuries happen at work. Please follow all necessary precautions while on the job. Everyone says, "This can't happen to me." Use common sense. If you say to yourself, "I shouldn't be doing this," you are probably right. Don't take the risk.

ALZHEIMER'S

Alzheimer's affects approximately one in ten people in this country over the age of 65 and about one in two over the age of 85. However, this isn't the case everywhere. Elderly villagers in India have the lowest rates of Alzheimer's in the world and scientists are starting to suspect why. They think it's connected to their high consumption of curcumin. Curcumin is a compound found in the spice turmeric. Curcumin has powerful antioxidant and anti-inflammatory properties and Indians eat turmeric with most every meal. Animal studies are starting to confirm the connection. Also, older adults whose total folate intake is at or above the recommended daily guidelines can cut their risk of developing Alzheimer's by as much as 50 percent. Folate is found in leafy green vegetables, broccoli, oranges, asparagus, and many other foods.

Prescription drugs can contribute to Alzheimer's, especially with long-term usage. The list of medications that can lead to dementia is longer that you would think and includes drugs use to treat allergies, anxiety, heart problems and inflammation. This is why changing your lifestyle and avoiding drug use should be your first choice. Discuss the options with your doctor while also doing your own research at www.drugs.com.

Centenarian Secret

One-third of centenarians have had no significant changes in their thinking abilities. High homocysteine levels, on the other hand, may contribute to dementia or Alzheimer's. However, homocysteine levels may be reduced by taking folate with vitamins B6 and B12. You can further reduce your risk of Alzheimer's by maintaining a healthy cardiovascular system. Statin drugs are suspected to contribute to Alzheimer's. Talk to your doctor about changing your lifestyle before making these drugs a life sentence.

STROKE

Strokes can be debilitating, and they are also preventable. Over time, sufferers often develop symptoms of dementia. A small stroke can also masquerade as dementia. The guidelines for reducing your chances of a stroke are similar to those for heart disease. Work to keep your blood pressure within normal ranges. If it's elevated, get in shape by making the self-care and health care changes you know you need to make. You can't control some risks, such as family history, age, and race, but you can control the leading cause—an unhealthy lifestyle and high blood pressure—as well as contributing factors such as smoking and diabetes. Follow the diet of populations around the world that tend not to have strokes. This means a low-calorie, plant-based diet that is high in unrefined carbohydrates. Additional preventive measures include:

- Lower your intake of cholesterol and saturated fat.
- Don't smoke.
- Control diabetes.
- Maintain a healthy weight.
- Get at least 30 minutes of exercise three to five days per week.
- Manage stress.

- Limit alcohol consumption.
- Keep your spine and nervous system healthy and functioning without interference
- Implement the Health Care Hierarchy of The 100 Year Life-style in the next chapter.

Chiropractic care is extremely safe. In a recent interview, Jean-Marc Slak, DC, Chairman of the Massachusetts Board of Registration of Chiropractors stated, "After several years as a member of my State's Regulatory Board, in charge of protecting the public, making rules, and enforcing the laws, I have made some revealing observations about the reality of chiropractic in our society. In my State, at least 50,000,000 visits to chiropractors have taken place during my tenure (2,500 chiropractors seeing 100 visits per week – a conservative estimate – 50 weeks a year for 4 years). Out of this 50 million visits sample, a single instance of sexual misconduct occurred (1 in 50 million!), only a dozen people reported minor injury (1 in about 4.1 million) and very few cases of fraudulent billing were discovered. Chiropractors offer an astonishingly safe service assisting millions of people."

CHRONIC OBSTRUCTIVE PULMONARY DISEASE (COPD)

Chronic obstructive pulmonary disease (COPD) is a group of chronic lung conditions that includes emphysema and chronic bronchitis. Once again, they are also preventable. Such lung conditions makes it more and more difficult to breathe and breathing is one of those very important functions that you want to excel at for a lifetime. COPD is strongly associated with lung cancer, the leading cause of cancer deaths. The main cause is smoking. Studies show that few centenarians have a substantial history of smoking. In fact, very few have ever smoked. Another risk factor is exposure to indoor or outdoor pollutants. Nearly 20 percent of cases are also attributed to work-related exposure.

Some preventive measures you can take:

- Don't smoke.
- Avoid secondhand smoke.
- Minimize exposure to workplace chemicals.
- Use air filters in your home and work to ensure that you breathe the cleanest air possible, especially if you live in a city where smog alerts are common.
- Keep your spine and nervous system healthy and functioning without interference.
- Implement the Health Care Hierarchy of The 100 Year Lifestyle in the next chapter.

Pneumonia and influenza are especially life-threatening to people whose lungs have already been damaged by COPD, asthma, or smoking. The risk of death from pneumonia or influenza is also higher among people with heart disease, diabetes, or a weakened immune system due to AIDS or immunosuppressive drugs. You can keep your resistance high with exercise, stress-free living, a healthy diet, keeping your spine, nerve, and immune system functioning properly and breathing clean air.

DIABETES

There are several types of diabetes. All of them can be managed and research shows that type 2 diabetes is also preventable or can be postponed for many years. It results when your body no longer produces insulin correctly. This is the most common form of diabetes. Approximately 18.2 percent of Americans have diabetes and almost one-third of those people don't know they have it. An additional 41 million people have prediabetes—or impaired glucose tolerance.

Excess body fat, especially around the middle, is an important risk factor for diabetes. About 80 percent of people who have the disease are either overweight or obese. The diabetes complications most likely to be fatal are heart disease and stroke, which occur at two' to four times the average rate in people with diabetes. People with diabetes haven't benefited as much from recent advances in heart disease treatment as have people without diabetes. During the past 30 years, deaths from heart disease have fallen 36 percent in men without diabetes, as compared with only 13 percent in men who have diabetes. Some preventive measures you can take:

- Maintain a healthy weight.
- Eat a varied diet, rich in fruits, vegetables, and low-fat foods.
- Get at least 30 minutes of exercise three to five days per week.
- Get your fasting blood sugar level checked periodically.
- Know your family's diabetes history and discuss it with your doctor.
- Keep your spine and nervous system healthy and functioning without interference.
- Implement the Health Care Hierarchy of The 100 Year Lifestyle in the next chapter.

SUICIDE

In 2010, 38,364 men committed suicide. Men commit suicide four times as often as women do. Depression—which is estimated to affect 7 percent of men in any given year—is an important risk factor for suicide. But male depression may be underdiagnosed, partly because men are less likely than women are to seek treatment for it or perform the proactive self-care or health care strategies for prevention. In addition, men don't always develop standard symptoms such as sadness, feelings of worthlessness, and excessive guilt. Instead, they may be more likely to complain of fatigue, irritability, sleep disturbances, and loss of interest in work or hobbies. Substance abuse of prescription or recreational drugs—which is more common in men—can mask depression and make it more difficult to diagnose. People at risk of suicide may:

- Be depressed, moody, socially withdrawn, or aggressive
- Have suffered a recent life crisis
- Show changes in personality
- Feel worthless
- Abuse alcohol or drugs
- Have frequent thoughts about death
- Talk about death and self-destruction

If you find yourself avoiding others, feeling hostile and worthless, thinking about death and using alcohol and drugs to numb your pain, you are in a destructive energy pattern. Shift yourself by changing your Dominant Energy Pattern on your own, or if you need to, with the help of a professional. In an urgent situation, an emergency room or crisis center can help. Friends or family members may be the first to notice your uncharacteristic behavior. Take their advice and seek help.

FDA MISSION AND SCIENCE AT RISK

Before you take another pill of any kind, you must read the 60 page report published by the FDA in 2007 entitled FDA Science and Mission at Risk, available at www.fda.gov. The following are quotes from the report:

1. "The FDA cannot fulfill its mission because its scientific base has eroded and its scientific organizational structure is weak."
2. "The FDA cannot fulfill its mission because its scientific workforce does not have sufficient capacity and capability."
3. The FDA cannot fulfill its mission because its information technology infrastructure is inadequate."
4. "The FDA does not have the capability to ensure the safety of food for the nation."
5. "The development of medical products based on 'new science' cannot be adequately regulated by the FDA."
6. "There is insufficient capacity in modeling, risk assessment, and analysis."
7. "The FDA science agenda lacks a coherent structure and vision, as well as effective coordination and prioritization."
8. "The FDA has substantial recruitment and retention challenges."
9. "The FDA has an inadequate and ineffective program for scientist performance."
10. "The FDA has not taken sufficient advantage of external and internal collaborations."
11. The FDA lacks the information science capability and information infrastructure to fulfill its regulatory mandate."
12. "The FDA cannot provide the information infrastructure support to regulate products based on new science."

A serious concern about drug testing is that it only takes about 8 years for a drug to be approved by the FDA. The side effects and the testing are not designed for long term usage. If you start taking a drug for a health problem at age 40 and it was only tested for 8 years, this takes you to age 48. If you continue for another 10, 20, or 40 years, you could be setting yourself up for severe consequences and side effects which may include heart attacks, strokes, kidney failure and dementia. Think about the drug ads you see on TV, hear on the radio or read in magazines. During the next TV commercial, close your eyes and listen to the severity and extent of the side effects that are being announced instead of watching the happy smiling people enjoying lavish vacations or dancing around in a beautiful green field. So many health problems and side effects can be avoided down the road if you are willing to adjust your lifestyle today.

KIDNEY DISEASE

Kidney failure, most often a complication of diabetes or high blood pressure, sends an estimated 400,000 Americans into crisis each year. Control of diabetes and high blood pressure can prevent or slow the progression of kidney disease. Another cause of kidney failure is overuse of medications such as NSAIDS (nonsteroidal anti-inflammatory drugs), such as ibuprofen (Advil, Motrin, etc.) that are toxic to the kidneys. Some preventive measures you can take:

- Drink plenty of fluids.
- Exercise regularly.
- Maintain your proper weight.
- Don't smoke.
- Get checked regularly for diabetes and high blood pressure.
- Make excellent self-care and drug-free health care choices whenever possible to prevent and minimize your need for both prescription and over-the-counter medication.
- Keep your spine and nervous system healthy and functioning without interference
- Implement the Health Care Hierarchy of The 100 Year Lifestyle in the next chapter.

CHRONIC LIVER DISEASE AND CIRRHOSIS

Cirrhosis is the tenth leading cause of death nationwide, causing approximately 30,000 deaths each year. The leading cause of liver disease, in general, is alcoholism, which takes a heavy toll on men in general. Men account for more than 70 percent of the 100,000 alcohol-attributable deaths that occur each year in the United States.

Other leading causes of chronic liver disease and cirrhosis include hepatitis B and C and certain inherited diseases such as hemochromatosis, in which abnormal amounts of iron accumulate in the liver. Nonalcoholic fatty liver disease, which is associated with obesity, also sometimes leads to cirrhosis. Some preventive measures you can take:

- Don't drink alcohol to excess.
- Take precautions when using hazardous chemicals.
- Practice safe sex.
- Don't inject street drugs.
- Make excellent self-care and drug-free health care choices whenever possible.
- Maintain a healthy weight.
- Keep your spine and nervous system healthy and functioning without interference
- Implement the Health Care Hierarchy of The 100 Year Lifestyle in the next chapter.

Write a New Family Tree
Gather health data on all of your immediate family members. For any members who have passed away, find out what they died from.
Your mother: _____
Your father: _____
Your father's parents: _____
Your mother's parents: _____
Your siblings: _____
Turn Over a New Leaf:
Since I have a family history of _____, _____
and _____, the healthy habits that I will begin
immediately are:
1._____
2._____
3._____
4._____
5._____

YOU DESERVE TO BE HEALTHY FOR A LIFETIME

Make your health a priority and keep yourself healthy for a lifetime. Understand the potential risks of your family history, but instead of worrying about them make lifestyle choices today, and every day, to support the quality of your longevity. Trust your body's ability to adapt to your environment and nurture its adaptability through your 100 Year Lifestyle choices. It will improve your life today and tomorrow. Educate yourself. Eat healthy foods, stay physically active, keep your spine and nervous system aligned and balanced with chiropractic Lifestyle Care, stay away from cigarettes, get regular checkups, and guard against accidents every day. By making this a way of life, you'll increase your chances of staying healthy and active beyond 100 years, or for however many years you have left.

Growing Concern With Every Shot
Contributed by Aryn Gabai, D.C.

There is a growing concern that one of the major threats to the development of healthy immune systems has been the increasing emphasis on artificial immunity through vaccines. As of 2010, the Center for Disease Control and Prevention in the United States was recommending 30 vaccinations before the age of 2 years old. At the same time, rates of asthma, autism, allergies, digestive disorders, autoimmune diseases, cancer, and many other chronic conditions are also rising. Many scientists, chiropractors, medical doctors and parents have become alarmed that this massive volume and combination of inoculations is jeopardizing the long-term health of individuals and future generations. In fact, according to the U.S. Department of Health and Human Services, over $2 Billion has already been paid to parents of vaccine-injured children. (1)

Japan, who has one of the highest life expectancy rates and lowest infant mortality rates, has had a voluntary vaccination policy since 1994. The US ranks 38 in life expectancy with a significantly higher infant mortality and has one of the most stringent mandatory vaccination policies in the world.(2)

A vaccine works by combining four major parts: the pathogen (bacteria or virus), an amplifier, a growth material and a stabilizer.

A very small amount of pathogen is not likely to cause an immune response from your body, so an amplifier called an adjuvant is added that chemically causes an immune system reaction that puts your body on the "highest threat level." With this type of stimulation, the immune cells become extremely reactive to anything that seems suspicious, whether it is the vaccine, pollen, a food or even normal human cells. In addition to these adjuvants, growth materials like egg yolk, rhesus monkey embryo and, in some vaccines, aborted human fetus cells are included as the liquid medium for the pathogen. (3) As these materials are injected at the same time as the adjuvants, they may cause an immune reaction. The final ingredient in a vaccine is a stabilizer like formaldehyde, a known cancer-causing agent for which there is no safe allowable limit for your body. (4)

These elements, introduced into your body through the process of a vaccination, can create hyper-stimulation, over-reactivity, and chemical toxicity. There is increasing doubt that the uncertain benefits of vaccines justify the risks.

Do your homework before you blindly get another shot or give one to your child. More information can be found on www.nvic.org or www.909shot.com .

References:
1. http://www.hrsa.gov/vaccinecompensation/statisticsreports.html
2. http://mothering.com/peggyomara/qpeditorials/voluntary-vaccines-in-japan
3. http://www.immunizationinfo.org/issues/vaccine-components/human-fetal-links-some-vaccines
4. http://www.cdc.gov/vaccines/vac-gen/additives.htm

Remember Life Changing Principle Number 2: Change comes one choice at a time. Think progress, not perfection. The Titration Principle can impact you negatively just as it can impact you positively. Smoking cigarettes is the most obvious and easy-to-embrace example of this concept. It is not the first cigarette that kills you. It is also not the last cigarette that kills you. It is the cumulative effect of all of the cigarettes over time that damages your lungs. Eventually this overwhelms the coping mechanisms of your body.

The same applies with obesity. Stop killing yourself with food. It is not an extra scoop of ice cream today that puts on the extra pounds. It's the accumulation of all the extra scoops over time. Are a few minutes of pleasure really worth it? Can you find healthier ways to treat yourself? Just like smoking, destructive eating patterns compromise our lives. Eating should always be a conscious choice. Try to make good choices every day. Remember: Think progress, not perfection. Choose with your ideal 100 Year Lifestyle in mind.

Without becoming another diet book, but understanding the importance of good nutrition, here is some basic eating advice. If you ever say to yourself, "I shouldn't be eating that," you shouldn't. If your Innate Intelligence tells you, "I should eat a salad today," you should listen. If your body is telling you it needs more fiber, vegetables, or protein, you should listen to it and give your body what it needs. Unfortunately, many of our destructive patterns have created confusion in our own minds. We don't know which voice to listen to. Begin to trust yourself again and connect to your inner voice. Healthy thoughts and actions lead to a healthy life and nobody is going to be able to make these choices for you. It's a step-by-step process, one choice at a time; think progress, not perfection.

Centenarian Secret
Lifelong vegetarians visit the hospital 22 percent less often than meat eaters, and have shorter stays. Vegetarians suffer 20 percent less premature mortality from all causes, compared with their meat-eating counterparts, according to the BBC online news service.

As I have traveled around the world, I have spoken to thousands of individuals who have made this shift in thinking. They know that their diet affects how they look and feel. They align their diets to those values. They have the same passion for food as everyone else. But instead of eating bacon with scrambled eggs in the mornings, they may have wild Alaskan sockeye salmon. Instead of cooking with margarine, they may use cold-pressed extra-virgin olive oil or butter. They have a healthy glow that comes from purified water throughout the day. They are eating with their 100 Year Lifestyle in mind. This benefits their lives today—they look and feel better—and it promotes longevity.

FUELING YOUR 100 YEAR LIFESTYLE

I would like to end this chapter with a short discussion of some superfoods that will help you "fuel" your 100 Year Lifestyle and stay healthy. First of all, some common mistakes: Women need protein and can age faster when they don't get enough of it. Protein is very important to men also. What you want to focus on are healthy protein sources. Always go organic. Although it's more expensive, you'll be glad you did. We will spend more time on this in the next chapter. Consider stocking your refrigerator with an organic chicken. You can cook the chicken and then make it into a light chicken salad for lunch or dinner, seasoning it with a golden onion—organic of course.

Miso is a great source of protein and can be prepared a variety of ways. Fish is also a great source of protein; however, as we all know, we must be careful with fish. A good selection is wild Alaskan sockeye salmon. Salmon is good for your body and skin. But you want to avoid farmed salmons. Did you know that farmed salmon is actually naturally gray in color? Yuck!

Some superfoods include:
- Wild salmon
- Blueberries
- Broccoli

- Tomatoes
- Miso
- Flaxseed
- Oats
- Strawberries
- Cantaloupe
- Garlic
- Beans
- Green tea

You have to be careful with fruits like strawberries. The best option may actually be to grow them at home since it is difficult to find organic strawberries. Plant a handful of strawberry plants, and they can easily fill up a garden bed in two to three years, with very little care. You will be pleased: nothing compares with the color and taste of a freshly picked, vine-ripened strawberry.

In fact, your best bet in many cases will be to grow your own fruits and vegetables during the warmer months. This is the purest form of organic eating. Easy things to grow include tomatoes, lettuce, cucumbers, and herbs like chives, parsley, and basil. Plant enough basil and you will have a steady supply all summer long of fresh pesto and greens to mix with your salads. In southern climates, chives and parsley keep producing all winter long.

What you can expect, when you eat this way, is a healthy glow and an overall sense of well-being. To the degree you can, try to get a little exercise after each meal. Especially as you age, this really helps your body utilize the nutrients you take in. You can practice true organic gardening by building or mixing garden beds with compost from the nursery. If you are making a garden bed, the mixture is one-third compost, one-third peat moss, and one-third perilite. Organic fertilizers are even available to nourish your soil and help your garden thrive.

TRUST YOUR INNATE INTELLIGENCE

The regenerative powers of your body are amazing. Have faith in it. Support it every day through your lifestyle choices, and stop killing yourself. If you have been in destructive energy patterns that have been deteriorating your health over time, you can turn things around with your next choice. If there is one thing I have learned after practicing for over 25 years and seeing thousands of patients with all types of health problems, it is that as long as you are alive and breathing you have the ability to heal, be healthy, and reach your potential. If you've accumulated damage to different parts of your body, you may need to adjust your lifestyle and design it to fit within your current capabilities. If running used to feel great and now it causes excruciating pain, switch to power walking, yoga, or riding a bicycle. Work with your chiropractor, health care and Crisis Care professionals to optimize your mind and body for your next phase of life. Take it on. It's not too late to make the changes you know you need to make. If you need support to make it happen, keep on reading and discover the abundance of resources available to you in the "Health Care Hierarchy" section coming up next.

THE 100 YEAR LIFESTYLE
ACTION PLAN FOR LASTING CHANGE

1. Stop killing yourself. If you are in a destructive energy pattern, stop now, and stay stopped with every choice from this moment on.

2. Trust your Innate Intelligence. As you begin to turn things around with your choices, your body and mind will strengthen. You will feel yourself getting sharper and younger in mind and body. This will give you the confidence to continue.

3. Take care of your original parts. Strengthen your weaknesses and adapt your activities to accommodate any areas of your body that are having challenges. Better to change your activities than drive your body parts into submission.

4. Don't just treat your crisis. Make self-care and health care a priority. Meet with the appropriate health care providers and develop a game plan to optimize your 100 Year Lifestyle while taking into consideration your personal history. Get a second or even a third opinion until the recommendations feel right in your gut, because once again, deep down, you know what it is best for you.

5. Also, learn your family history and become proactive with your health. Make self-care and health care a priority specifically as it relates to your family history.

6. Remember the three Life-Changing Principles. Change is easy; thinking about change is hard. It is much easier to make the changes for your quality of life, with every choice that supports your ideal 100 Year Lifestyle, than it is to continue on a destructive path and be forced to change by serious disease.

7. Get excited about what is possible from your current starting point. Look to make progress every day and be careful not to compare yourself to when you were 18 or 35. Get better and feel younger every day through your choices.

PART 4

The Health Care Hierarchy of The 100 Year Lifestyle

*When it comes to the old saying
'if it ain't broke don't fix it,'
we need to redefine broke.
When you are out
of balance, you're
broke.*

CHAPTER 7

CONSUMER-DRIVEN CHANGE IN THE HEALTH CARE INDUSTRY

Consumer demand is powerful and it is rapidly changing our health care industry. Consider for example, the way babies are born today. Many women opt for natural childbirth and have their husbands with them in the delivery rooms. This was not the case a generation or two ago when the 69 million baby boomers were born. Back then, fathers waited outside in reception rooms—pacing back and forth, smoking cigarettes, and waiting for the news that baby and mom made it through with all of their appendages intact. Today, smoking is taboo and childbirth is viewed as a much more intimate and natural experience. We are also seeing an increasing number of holistic birthing centers. Midwives and birthing coaches are often contracted to provide a natural form of support that is known to shorten labor times.

GOING ORGANIC

One of the biggest consumer-driven phenomena in recent history is the rise in popularity of organic foods. The rise in organic foods is a direct response to consumer demand. This healthy, chemical-free method of growing fruits and vegetables is now a $26 billion business worldwide and it is just beginning to gain momentum. North America has overtaken Europe as the largest market for organic foods. And the term "organic" doesn't apply only to fruits and veggies these days. We are also choosing organic meats, eggs, dairy products, oils, flours, and salad dressings. Organic yogurts and salad bars are making their way into the public schools, and farm to table restaurants featuring organic specialties are sprouting up in cities and towns nationwide. We are even starting to go organic when it comes to our pets. Organic pet foods are growing at nearly three times the rate of conventional foods even though they can be substantially more expensive.

There are more than 865 registered pesticides in the United States. Around 350 of those are used on the food we eat. Genetically modified foods, which are raising serious concerns because of their potentially severe health effects, are stocked on the grocery store shelves. There are 800 products on store shelves across the country—toothpaste, sodas, cookies, vitamins—that contain artificial sweeteners that are suspected of causing many symptoms from dizziness, to seizures, brain tumors, and migraines. Read the labels and avoid these foods at all costs.

Just a decade ago, eating organic often meant driving miles out of your way to a health food store. And it was hard to even find one. When I opened my first chiropractic office 25 years ago, there was only one within a five-mile radius—and that was in the heart of Atlanta, a big city. At the health food store, choices were limited and, well, not quite as vibrant or appealing as I would have liked. Battered and bruised apples were close to twice the price of conventional ones that were much shinier after being grown and treated with pesticides.

By comparison, organic today is mainstream. Whole Foods is revolutionizing the grocery business by mainstreaming healthier

food solutions. Whole Foods is considered high-end, but neverthe-
less consumers are flocking to their grocery stores in droves. Trader
Joe's, Fresh Market and other chains have emerged. This consumer
demand is driving competitors to begin stocking up on organic as
well. Advances in farming and distribution technology are helping
to make this possible. As the demand for organic foods continues
to increase, the competition and the pricing will make them more
affordable for all.

FROM ALTERNATIVE TREATMENTS TO MAINSTREAM HEALTH CARE LEADERS

We are also demanding more holistic care for our minds and
bodies. As a result, holistic health care options, Lifestyle Care in The
100 Year Lifestyle model, have become the first choice for millions
while traditional medical care is being reserved for severe Crisis
Care only and life-threatening emergencies.

The 100 Year Lifestyle is about so much more than cost-effec-
tive, high-tech crisis management. It is about exploring and expressing your full potential for a lifetime.

PUTTING THE "HEALTH" BACK IN HEALTH CARE

Taking control of our own health care—but more importantly,
our health—is an important aspect of The 100 Year Lifestyle. After
all, why get to 100, or even 50 years old, if you don't have the mind
and body to enjoy it? You'll want to optimize your health as a lifestyle to enjoy a great quality of life every day. But you may be asking
yourself how you can utilize all of the new information and resources
to make the most of it. How does it all fit together?

"Health care" as we know it today, in this country, is really Crisis
Care. Your medical physician is largely there to help you detect and

solve crises. In this respect, they are kind of like debt counselors. A debt counselor can play a vital role in helping you solve a financial crisis, get you out of trouble and back on track financially. But a debt counselor is not likely able to optimize the growth of your assets, your cash flow, or long-term financial planning.

Now, let's say you are in pursuit of financial freedom. How big a role will that debt counselor play toward your ultimate goal? A debt counselor might do a great job getting you on track if you're way off course managing your money. You might stabilize the foundation you need, but in order to build up sufficient reserves and become wealthy, you are going to have to master additional knowledge and utilize wealth-building resources. For example, you may need to speak with a financial planner and nurture this relationship as you grow. This type of specialist is not focused on bailing you out, but rather, they work with you on building up your reserves—in this case, cash reserves, cash flow and assets. This applies to your health as well, building your health reserves every day and avoiding "Crisis Care" for as long as possible throughout your lifetime.

How do you do this? How do you make sense of all of the information that is out there? How does it all fit together? And most importantly, how can you utilize the information to make the rest of your life the best? That is where the Health Care Hierarchy of The 100 Year Lifestyle comes into play. You'll be able to use this information to set priorities, goals, and take action to support the quality of life you desire and deserve.

THE HEALTH CARE HIERARCHY OF THE 100 YEAR LIFESTYLE

There are three levels to the Health Care Hierarchy of The 100 Year Lifestyle, as follows:

1. *Self-Care:* What you need to do for yourself to keep your mind, body, and spirit healthy and functioning at your highest level, which nobody else can do for you.

2. *Health Care:* What you need to do for yourself to keep your mind, body, and spirit healthy and functioning at your highest level—utilizing the skills of a trained health care professional.

3. *Crisis Care:* What you need to do for yourself to recover from an injury or illness that requires the support of a Crisis Care or health care specialist.

To live The 100 Year Lifestyle, healthy, it is important to make self-care and health care your priority. When you do, you will prevent the crisis for as long as possible.

This actually all goes back to what we discussed earlier in Life Changing Principle #2—the Titration Principle. When you focus on building health every day—the quality of your life will improve every day. Maybe this will require you to defer a little short-term pleasure for long-term benefit. On the upside, it's generally cheaper over time, less painful and much more fun to be healthy. But it requires you to be motivated by something greater than a crisis.

Identify the things you like doing in the realm of self-care and do them every day.

Live your ideal 100 Year lifestyle daily.

Everyone deserves to be healthy and express their full potential from the time they are born through their last breath of life. This includes you. This includes you. This includes your family. Living the Health Care Hierarchy and Philosophy of The 100 Year Lifestyle will improve your health dramatically.

Health Care Philosophy

Everyone deserves to be healthy and express their full potential from the time they are born through their last breath of life. This includes you! The Health Care Philosophy of The 100 Year Lifestyle states the following:

1.   Innate Intelligence

You have within you an Innate Intelligence. Present from the moment you were conceived, this Intelligence guides the processes in your body that turn food into cells, eliminates waste products, coordinates muscle contraction and communicates with or without your conscious thought to every cell, tissue and organ of your body via your nervous system. As long as there is no interference to this system, you have the capability to heal, feel great, be healthy and function well for a lifetime. Nurture this Intelligence for the development of your human potential and you will set personal records in all areas of your life.

2.   Interference

Unfortunately, there can be interference to the communication and expression of this Intelligence within your body. This interference causes dis-ease, weakness, and imbalances with your nervous system that can cause all types of immediate health problems. Or, this interference can lie dormant and asymptomatic for decades, leading to severe health conditions, chronic pain, deterioration and disease down the road.

Nerve interference in the spine is called a vertebral subluxation. Lifestyle interference is a result of poor health habits such as overeating, poor nutrition, excessive drinking, taking prescription or non-prescription drugs, or sitting too much. Environmental interference is caused by toxicity from air, food, water, or chemicals, as well as accidents or natural disasters. All three types of interference can cause pressure in your spine and nervous system and affect your health on every level.

3.   Adjustments

Remove the interference from your body through adjustments to your environment, lifestyle, spine and nervous system so that your body can heal itself and function at optimum health and peak performance levels for a lifetime.

Visit our website www100yearlifestyle.com

Like our Fan page www.facebook.com/100yearlifestyle

Watch our YouTube Channel http://www.youtube.com/user/100yearlifestyle

CHAPTER 8

SELF-CARE: MAKING YOUR QUALITY OF LIFE A PRIORITY

Self-care is about taking care of yourself, your mind, body, and spirit. It's about you being responsible for you and doing the things that you know are good for you. Good self-care works with your body's natural ability to be healthy, adapt to stress, maintain strong resistance to disease, and stay in balance. Be good to yourself and make self-care your lifestyle.

This includes eating the foods that you know are right for you, drinking clean water and breathing clean air. Good self-care includes managing your physique, your energy, and your stress level, and participating in activities that are healthy. Have fun doing things that make you feel strong and vibrant every day.

Many people think that self-care is hard. But this isn't true. Self-care isn't hard—it's actually easy. What *can* be hard is changing your pattern from a destructive or complacent one to a Human Potential Pattern. Remember Life Changing Principle Number 1: change is easy—thinking about change is hard. Being on the fence is hard. Going back and forth from "should I?" to "shouldn't I?" is hard. The reality is that roller coaster crisis management is the hardest of all.

Self-care requires you to make time for you and can be "time consuming." The truth is you are spending the time anyway so why not spend it with your ideal 100 Year Lifestyle in mind? Great self-care will give you more time by enhancing your energy, strength, and focus. You'll need less sleep, have more energy, more fun and more personal confidence. If not now, when?

Personal Fitness or Cardiac Rehab?

What is the difference between being on a personal fitness program and going to a cardiac rehabilitation program? The answer is quite simple "timing".

Personal fitness is a key element of living The 100 Year Lifestyle while cardiac rehab happens after you have had a heart attack. Otherwise, the procedures of each are similar. Many people who are into personal fitness wear a heart monitor to track their results.

During cardiac rehab, the cardiac specialists hook you up to a more sophisticated heart monitor to minimize your risks and their liability. At some point you are either going to choose to make fitness a part of a proactive healthy lifestyle or be forced into fitness because of a life-threatening crisis. What is your primary motivation? Crisis or quality of life? Make a conscious choice right now!

Self-care is about the choices you make every day—thinking healthy thoughts, cultivating high-quality relationships, meditating, and maintaining an exercise routine. If taking care of yourself has not been your norm, it's time to start now before a crisis occurs. This may mean making some positive changes that impact your life one choice at a time. One healthy food choice will lead to another. A good workout will inspire you to have another one. Be consistent and eventually you'll feel that you've found your path and your results will motivate you to get to the next level. Do the right things and eventually they will become your new human potential pattern.

Constantly explore new avenues to keep your self-care fun and interesting. If you love yoga, try hot yoga—a growing trend that detoxifies the body. Other popular self-care activities include strength training, sports, gardening, running, aerobics, meditating, attending seminars, listening to music or audio books, taking vacations, swimming, sailing, spiritual retreats, spas, reading, and Pilates to name a few. You'll know your routine is working for you when it doesn't feel like work. It should be fun and refresh your mind, body, and spirit. You will refine your ideal self-care routine over time.

LIVE LONG AND STRONG EXERCISE
The self-care that I want to incorporate into my lifestyle immediately is:
1. _____
2. _____
3. _____
4. _____
5. _____

In addition to keeping your body and mind strong, self-care keeps your immune system strong so that your resistance to infections stays high. Maintaining your resistance is a key component of The 100 Year Lifestyle. Have you ever noticed that healthy people are less likely to get sick than sickly people? Sickly people attract disease. Their bodies become better hosts for diseases to flourish. Keeping yourself healthy with the discipline of great self-care and health care is a much better option. This chapter will cover in detail some of the Self-Care practices you can adopt.

GET YOUR ESS IN SHAPE®

Regular exercise is an important part of self-care and nobody can do it for you. It keeps our minds and bodies healthy. *The 100 Year Lifestyle Workout* became the #1 Bestseller in its category on Amazon when it was released. It is designed to help people at any level and any age to make the fitness part of their self-care fun and exciting whether they are beginners, intermediates or high level athletes. If you are not currently exercising, are you waiting to be forced into it by a crisis? If you are already exercising, take it to the next level and Get Your ESS in Shape. Your ESS is made up of your:

- Endurance
- Strength
- Structure

> The 100 Year Lifestyle Workout book has great exercise programs for beginner, intermediate and advanced exercisers. Getting your ESS in Shape is important for your health, quality of life and longevity.

ENDURANCE

Would you trust your body to take you on a long-distance trek in an emergency? If you had to count on your body to save a loved one who needed you to be physically strong, would you be able to? If you had to run away to escape danger, could you? Your endurance is important for all these activities, and it is important for longevity.

If you have good endurance, you will enjoy a great sense of stamina and activity now and while you age. Your energy will be high and you will feel like doing things. You will not be left home alone while your partner goes off to experience the world. You can increase your stamina through cardiovascular, aerobic, exercise that strengthens your heart, burns calories, and increases your energy. Running, cycling, swimming, and power walking are just a few examples of types of exercise that will increase your endurance.

Centenarian Secret

Set goals for your endurance and continue to challenge yourself. Increase the length of time that you spend doing cardiovascular exercise by 10 percent each month for the next three months and increase your intensity as well. If you are not an experienced exerciser, make sure you consult with a certified personal trainer who can customize an endurance plan especially for you.

If you already have arthritic or prearthritic conditions, low-impact exercise becomes more and more important as you age. This is why equipment such as elliptical machines, bicycles, rowing machines, and stair-steppers are so popular with people over 50 years of age. They let you exercise your cardiovascular and muscular systems without pounding your joints and your spine.

Endurance training is very important to keep your heart and lungs healthy, eliminate stress, and strengthen your immune system. Always exercise with a heart monitor to maximize your results and achieve your goals, while also ensuring that you exercise safely within the normal ranges for your age.

Calculate your exercise target heart rate by age

Age:	20	30	40	50	60	70
65 percent	130	123	117	110	104	97
85 percent	170	161	153	144	136	127

Organizations like NASM, The National Academy of Sports Medicine and The American Council on Exercise have created guidelines for people up to the age of seventy. With The 100 Year Lifestyle, you and I will create the standard for future generations.

STRENGTH

Strength training is also important for healthy aging because you are going to want and need your strong muscles to keep you confident and maintain your independence as you age. We've all seen an older person struggle to get out of a chair. If you have good strength, you are more likely to remain self-sufficient and independent. Strength training can be done through weights, yoga, and Pilates. When you set goals for strength training and continually strive to achieve them, you will be excited to see that your strength can increase as you age. Your muscles can stay strong and defined. The sagging skin and muscles often come from not keeping your body toned through strength-training exercise.

If you are already an experienced strength trainer and have a routine already, shake it up a little bit. Try increasing your weight by 10 percent to 20 percent. Get somebody to spot you if necessary and try to squeeze out a few more reps. Vary your exercises on each body part. Companies like CrossFit have become extremely popular because they set up your routines and vary them for you. The workout program at www.100yearlifestyle.com does it for you as well. Work out with a partner and challenge each other. You will begin to see a better result. Always maintain good posture when you strength train to ensure that your spine stays healthy during your training.

We've all heard the expression "if you don't use it, you lose it." This is absolutely true with your strength. Once again, if you have not been actively involved in a strength-training program, consult with a health professional and customize your program.

STRUCTURE

In countries where longevity is much higher than the U.S., posture and the spine are a very high priority. Your structure includes your body shape and physical frame. Keeping your structure, spine and nervous system in shape will keep you looking good and help to prevent injuries while you exercise. You will be healthier on every level.

How is your structure now? Is your waist the size that you desire it to be? How about your arms, your chest, and your legs? Have you measured yourself lately and set goals for your structure so that it is in the shape you desire over your lifetime? You can measure your structure with your eyes at first and decide how you want to change your shape, or get a tape measure and record your specific measurements. This will give you a starting point for goals that you want to set. Measure your neck, biceps, chest, waist, thighs, and calves. If you do not include your structure in your fitness regime, you will find that you start exercising to get in shape, but your shape stays the same as it was before, only you will be a smaller version of yourself. If you are pear shaped and just start doing endurance training, you will become a smaller pear. To truly jump-start you in the direction of your ideal shape, visit a fitness professional and have them develop a program that is personal for you.

Another important part of your structure is your spine, nervous system and posture. A simple way to test its condition is by doing a weight balance test. Rather than stepping on one scale and measuring your weight, you can use two scales and put one foot on each scale. Have somebody else read the numbers for you because if you look down you will tend to sway and throw off your readings. If you are more than three pounds difference on one side of your body compared to the other, your body is out of balance and you are overdue for a chiropractic check-up. You will be putting unnecessary strain on your structure, spine and nervous system when you exercise and run the risk of injury.

Evaluate your posture. Take the Posture Test on www.100 YearLifestyle.com or on The 100 Year Lifestyle Fan Page on Facebook.

When I was in full-time practice I used to attend a lot of 5K and 10K road races and volunteer my time to examine the runners. I couldn't believe how many of them were out of balance. It was very common to see people that were ten pounds heavier on one side of their body compared to the other. That's like carrying a bowling ball on one of your hips. Over time this can lead to repetitive strain injuries and serious spinal problems that are completely preventable if you just keep your structure, spine and nervous system in balance. I used to love to see people's posture change and their bodies get back into balance within a few adjustments and have them rave about the improvements to their running with their Lifestyle Care. Many professional athletes incorporate chiropractic adjustments into their regular training routine for this reason, as well as to improve recovery time between games and practices, and to speed the healing time of injuries. You can read some of their stories in *The 100 Year Lifestyle Workout*.

Balance is crucial to being able to enjoy exercise for the long haul. Weight and postural balance are an important part of healthy exercise and properly caring for your physical structure.

If you really want to get your ESS in shape, make the commitment to see your fitness professional today or design a fitness program at www.100yearlifestyle.com and click on "Get Your ESS in Shape."

LIVE LONG AND STRONG
100 Year Lifestyle Fitness Goal: Get Your ESS in Shape
Endurance: Do at least 30 minutes of cardiovascular training three to five times a week. Exercise with a heart monitor and monitor your baseline. Get a personal trainer or other health professional to monitor your progress and get you started on the right track.
Strength: Evaluate the strength of your major muscle groups, including your chest muscles, back muscles, arms, legs and core. Set goals for building your strength in each of these areas and get a personal trainer or other health professional to get you started on the right track.
Structure: Measure your neck, chest, waist, hips, and thighs. Evaluate your posture and your weight balance. Set goals for your shape in each of these areas and get a chiropractor, personal trainer, or other health professional to start you on the right track.
Customize an exercise program for yourself and set goals at www.100yearlifestyle.com. Keep yourself active, strong, and balanced as you age.

Also, pay attention to your chairs, mattresses, and bedding, particularly as you age. You want them to support your spine. They should support the natural curvature of your neck and back. You will start to feel like you are old when you start to feel old physically because your body gets stiff, sore, and tight. It's hard to believe, but we actually spend a third of our lives lying down—sleeping. If you sleep eight hours a night and you live to 100, you will spend 33 years in a bed. And if you are like many of us and have a desk job, you probably spend close to another third sitting. This is why ergonomic chairs that support your body properly are an important component of self-care.

A good bed will not be too hard, and it won't be too soft either. Like the porridge in the "Goldilocks and the Three Bears" nursery rhyme, it will be just right. Many bed manufacturers today have technology that can measure the pressure in your spine when you lay down on a bed to see how it fits your body. Using a pillow that supports the natural curve in your neck is also important to ensure its stability and to keep pressure off of your nerves. Your chiropractor can perform an examination to show you how your neck is positioned so that you can make the appropriate choices for your long-term well-being. You should be able to personalize your side of the bed so that you and your spouse can both enjoy the refreshing feeling of a good night's sleep, consistently.

Ergonomically designed chairs, computer workstations, and work platforms are important to ensure that you don't injure yourself on the job. When I got into practice in the mid-eighties, the science of ergonomics was barely known in the work world. Today, it is hard to find a responsible company that does not take ergonomics into consideration for their employees. Be responsible for your own safety, however, with good self-care on the job. If you sit at a computer for any length of time, make sure that your knees are at a 90-degree bend and your feet are flat on the floor or slightly elevated. Make sure your spine is straight and your shoulders hang comfortably, keeping your lower arms parallel to the floor.

Always lift with your legs and not your back. Statistics show that 80 percent of the population will have a severe episode of back pain at some point in their life. Good self-care and health care choices will keep you healthy and prevent you from feeling old before your time.

PROVIDE YOUR BODY WITH EXTRA PROTECTION FROM HARMFUL SUBSTANCES

The air in your environment will be inside your body when you breathe. The water in your home and the food you eat will also be ingested and become a part of your body. If you want to help your body stay healthy, keep the air and water clean.

USE AIR AND WATER FILTERS

A few years ago my son had some friends over to the house for a party and since it was winter, I thought it would be nice to light up the fireplace. Little did I know that some creature had built a nest in our chimney, and before we knew it the entire house was filled up with smoke. We had to evacuate the house, open all the windows and doors, and let the house air out.

When all the visible smoke had cleared, we went back inside and unfortunately, the smell was very present and we could feel the ill effects by the next morning. I went out and bought two air filters and ran them in the house the next few days, and I was thrilled at how well they worked. I stopped taking the air that we breathe for granted after that episode.

Air pollution is a problem in the United States. Chemical trails can be seen across the skies which create an eyesore on the beautiful blue backdrop. Use of air filters, washing your bedding often, and following smog alerts can make a difference. Avoid exercising outside on smoggy days, and consider cutting back on all the lawn chemical treatments. In many parts of the country, having a lawn that looks "golf-course good" is the new standard. Unfortunately, many of those chemicals are highly toxic. Consider organic alternatives.

Airborne toxins affect our health in a variety of ways and come in a variety of forms:

- Ozone: The major component of smog and most pervasive air pollutants, this poisonous allotrope can cause severe coughing, shortness of breath, pained breathing, lung and eye irritation, and greater susceptibility to pneumonia, bronchitis, and other respiratory illnesses.
- Dioxin: One of the most potent animal carcinogens ever tested, dioxin can cause severe weight loss, liver problems, kidney problems, birth defects, and death.
- Nitrogen Oxide: a major component of acid rain. It can damage lung tissue.
- Volatile Organic Compounds: These compounds are generated by power plants, motor vehicles, and waste combustors. They are associated with cancer, and neurological and reproductive problems.
- Natural Allergens: Allergens (like pollen and fungal spores) can contribute to increased rates of asthma, allergies, and respiratory conditions when your body is not functioning properly.

DRINK PURIFIED WATER

One of the very best things you can do for your health is to drink purified water. This means investing in water filters for your home and investing in highly purified bottled water. Sure, a gallon of clean water can be even more expensive than a gallon of gasoline, which is a shame—but it's worth it.

Centenarian Secret
According to UNICEF, *4,000 children die each day from disease attributable to unsafe drinking water, deplorable sanitation and poor hygiene.*

In the United States, pesticides, fertilizers, animal excrement, bacteria, oil spills, radiation, and other toxins also make their way into our ground water supply. In fact, about one-third of the U.S. drinking water supply tested recently by the Natural Resources Defense Council showed the presence of arsenic, bacteria, organic chemicals, and other substances. Cumulative exposure can cause cancer as well as vomiting, abdominal pain, and other problems. The quick and easy disposal of waste in this country—again, another short-term gain—threatens our collective long-term health.

AVOID TOXIC CHEMICALS

Your body is a collection of chemicals—from the hydrochloric acid that breaks down the food in your stomach to the oxygen that converts it into energy and the minerals that nourish your organs. When these processes are balanced and regulated properly by your nervous system, your body has the ability to minimize the effects of these toxins and fight off disease. Unfortunately, the acid, pH, iron, and other chemical levels in your body can become out of balance, negatively affecting your health. External irritants can overwhelm your body's natural coping mechanisms, especially if your body is out of balance to begin with. Many of the irritants and toxins are invisible, and we really don't choose to have them enter our bodies. Keeping your body strong and healthy with great self-care and health care will keep your body in the best condition possible to resist their negative impact and cleanse them from your system.

Centenarian Secret

According to the *Journal of American Medicine*, tobacco use killed more people in the United States in 2000 than any other substance. Approximately 435,000 people died from the cumulative effects of tobacco exposure, 85,000 died from alcohol-related illnesses, and another 17,000 from using illegal drugs.

Tobacco, alcohol, and illegal drugs all cause chemical toxicity that can interfere with the body's natural ability to be healthy. But so do many over-the-counter and prescription drugs. Every year, more than 2 million people experience adverse drug reactions from properly prescribed medications. Nearly 100,000 die from chemical reactions to ordinary medicines you might find in your own bathroom cabinet. One of the reasons why this is so prevalent today is that we believe a magic pill exists for all of our ills. Too often, we reach for medications to dull our pain, alter our children's behavior, increase our libido, or enhance our athletic prowess without a second thought as to their side effects. The problem is that we are often risking our long-term health for short-term relief.

Over-the-counter and prescription drugs can cause adverse side effects like organ deterioration, organ dysfunction, and possible death. Many people have the notion that over-the-counter medications must be completely safe, but in reality, we all need to use caution when taking any type of medicine. Take it only as a last resort and when other holistic solutions have been ineffective. Beware of their side effects, study the contraindications, and don't exceed the recommended dosage. Consider holistic self-care and health care options whenever possible and use medications only as a last resort.

Centenarian Secret
According to the Centers for Education and Research on Therapeutics, over 2 million people experience serious adverse drug reactions each year. Also, according to the National Center for Immunization and Respiratory Diseases, tens of millions of antibiotic prescriptions are written for viral infections that they are unable to treat.

Continuous exposure to any type of toxin will force your body into a chronic stress reaction—draining your energy over time and distracting your body from its Innate goals. As it moves into and stays in a reactive mode in an attempt to ward off the side effects of these toxins, your body can go into survival and shut down. Why not prevent this and keep it clean and healthy.

STRESS LESS. LIVE MORE.

Managing stress is a key component of The 100 Year Lifestyle. A benefit of our extended life span is the knowledge that we can survive the challenges that life throws our way.

Your body is adaptable with remarkable capacities to heal. Empower it as much as you can through your lifestyle. This way, you'll be prepared to handle everything the future brings—which you can count on as being a mixture of good and bad—joyous times and challenging ones. Either way you'll be ready. Knowing that you have survived thus far will keep you from suffering extreme ups and downs that can increase your stress unnecessarily. Decide whether you will be the kind of person that makes a situation better or worse when you are exposed to a challenge. Having faith that you will make the most of every situation will certainly bring you through the challenging times and help you come out on top.

Think about all the events or issues that you have worried about over the years. Isn't it great to know that you have come through them all with the wisdom and confidence that you will survive and maybe even come out better from the experience? Combining this wisdom and maturity with the fully developed talents and the inner knowledge about yourself is another aspect of The 100 Year Lifestyle that is exciting and can help us to manage stress more effectively, and the benefits are many. I'll discuss methods that can be used to achieve these benefits in the following sections.

Stress Less. Live More.™
Many of The 100 Year Lifestyle Licensed Affiliate chiropractors deliver inspiring Stress Less. Live More. educational programs to companies, schools, organizations and associations. The resources for this program are outstanding. Find a licensed Affiliate in your area at www.100yearlifestyle.com.

MEDITATION

You can achieve a reduced stress level through practices like meditation. Meditation focuses your thoughts, produces a sense of calmness in your mind and body, and can strengthen your coping mechanisms in a crisis. Meditation requires regular practice—generally, once or twice a day for 20 to 30 minutes is sufficient. When you meditate, you are fully alert but you are not focused on the outside world. Instead, you cultivate inner awareness. You get to this state by focusing your mind on one thing—your breath, a single word, or an inspirational passage. Meditation is focused concentration and can even be done while exercising.

The best time to meditate is when you are free from distraction. This means when you are feeling fresh, comfortable, and relaxed. It can be a great way to start, break up, or end your day. It is often recommended that you stretch before you meditate, then take a seated position and assume a chosen meditation posture. This may be sitting cross-legged on the floor, or sitting up straight in a chair. You can also meditate lying flat on your back with your palms facing up. Close your eyes. Start to breathe in and breathe out—slowly and deeply. Count to seven or eight on each inhale and then again on each exhale. Make sure that you have good posture if you are sitting. Focusing on your breath is generally sufficient for producing a meditative state—although if you are a beginner, it may take some practice. If you are just getting started, you may consider buying some meditation guides. There are many excellent books, audios and videos to choose from.

YOGA

The best way to get acquainted with yoga is by trying out some classes and picking up an issue of one of the many excellent yoga magazines on bookshelves everywhere. There are myriad videos and DVDs available. However, you need to get a sense of the industry to find the levels, practices, and instructors that work for you. Yoga quiets the mind, improves concentration, stretches the muscles, builds strength and even massages internal organs. When you leave a good yoga class, you will feel like are glowing.

A good yoga instructor will gently guide you toward achieving optimal postures. A great yoga instructor will also focus on creating an optimal setting for your instruction. They know that you should feel relaxed and safe. Many instructors will dim the lights and use candles. They will carefully choose their music before each class. Their voices should be calming and nurturing. Yoga, along with all of the self-care and health care strategies discussed here, can make you feel younger and healthier within just a few weeks.

> **Centenarian Secret**
> Excessive stress shortens our lives, leads to chronic health problems, and also negatively impacts our relationships, work, and quality of life. Should you have something routinely stressing you right now, it is time for you to Stress Less. Live More. Make a choice to implement one of the suggestions in this chapter right now.

RETREATS

Self-care is about nurturing and nourishing your mind, body, and spirit. There are countless ways to do this. The important thing is that you choose activities that you enjoy doing and that you do them regularly. You might consider exploring new ideas at a spa. High-quality spas are all about great self-care and they will expose you to so many options to choose from. You'll learn meditation, chi gong, tai chi, power walking meditation, and yoga. For a super dose of self-care, spas are a superb solution. They remove you from your daily stresses and catapult you into the ultimate self-care experience. If you have never been to a spa that is completely dedicated to your self-care—with on-site health care providers whose purpose is to help you remove every ounce of stress from your body—you are really missing out. Everyone should go to a spa for at least one three-day weekend a year to break away and rejuvenate the spirit. If your finances permit (see Financing Your 100 Year Lifestyle later in the book), visit a spa at least once a quarter. The top spas around the world not only rejuvenate your mind, body, and spirit, but they also educate you on how to bring The 100 Year Lifestyle principles home with you.

As I travel around the world teaching these concepts to companies, health conscious individuals, chiropractors and other health care providers, I have noticed over the past few years how hotel chains have incorporated self-care amenities into their basic packages. In an effort to improve customer loyalty, the Starwood Hotel chain has upgraded to the Heavenly Bed and Westin Workouts powered by Reebok. Marriott just introduced Revive, their bed and relaxation system, and Hyatt and all of the other quality hotel chains are also upgrading their self-care systems to keep up and maintain their share of the market. They realize that the best way for them to care for their customers is to provide them with quality self-care resources while they are on the road away from home. While spas used to be, and still can be, exclusive for the rich and famous, spa facilities are available at nearly all hotel chains and the pricing for their services is comparable.

KEEP AN EYE ON YOUR SELF-CARE

How do you know if you are letting your self-care slip? You are probably overweight, overstressed, and are not getting enough rest. You are probably eating too much fast food and not taking time to balance your life. You are motivated by crisis and you only take care of yourself when you feel pain or you get sick. You find yourself on a crisis roller coaster, living from one challenge to the next, defining your life by these crises. You may even find yourself telling these crisis stories over and over and over again to your family and friends. Maybe you are taking constant trips to the drugstore, trying to mask symptoms rather than making trips to the gym, taking walks, visiting your local health food store or visiting your chiropractor for Lifestyle Care.

Creating your own personal human potential pattern for your self-care and health care will help you ensure the highest quality of life you desire and deserve.

CHAPTER 9

HEALTH CARE: BUILDING A QUALITY OF LIFE HEALTH CARE TEAM

Health care in The 100 Year Lifestyle model is a proactive way to keep your body and mind as healthy as possible and express your full potential for a lifetime. Health care is the care you cannot provide for yourself. It is necessary to keep your body balanced, aligned, stress free, and better able to resist the challenges of your environment. Just like you cannot do surgery on yourself in times of a crisis, there are many aspects of health care that are necessary to keep you functioning at your highest level that you cannot do for yourself.

As an example of health care, you cannot adjust your own spine, but your chiropractor can, which helps you keep your spine and nervous system healthy throughout your lifetime. You cannot massage yourself, but massage is important to keep your muscles and your lymphatic system healthy and to eliminate the accumulation of stress from your body. There are also times when you have difficulty thinking clearly about things—when it would be helpful to talk with a life coach, therapist, or a counselor. Maybe you've leveled off on the results you are getting from your exercise program, so you decide to consult with a personal trainer. Or it could be that you are having a difficult time with your diet and you would benefit from consulting a nutritionist. Building a health care team will help keep you in the best shape of your life.

TAKE CARE OF YOUR MIND AND BODY

In my chiropractic practice, I found that people who are committed to a Human Potential Pattern of self-care and health care almost always respond better when they are faced with a crisis. For example, I worked with a family that had a couple of severe health issues. The mother had recurring migraine headaches and one of her children had juvenile rheumatoid arthritis. Within a month of beginning their chiropractic Crisis Care, both the mom and daughter felt much better. Through the educational program on The 100 Year Lifestyle we provided, they began making healthier choices overall. They continued with their care through the Critical Transition to Lifestyle Care. Over time, their bodies began to heal and function much better on every level. The mother told me that she felt better than she had in years. Her daughter no longer needed the drugs that were beginning to cause severe side effects. She was back on the swim team and they were ecstatic about her health.

Her husband, however, did not share in her joy. While he was glad that everyone was feeling better, he was not supportive of the new health care routines. He was strictly motivated by crisis and did not see the value of self-care and ongoing Lifestyle Care. Unfortunately, one day the family was involved in a car accident. The entire family was in the car and experienced the same impact. They were all injured in similar ways, feeling the effects of the whiplash, but it was the husband who took the longest to recover. The rest of the family healed within a week while his recovery took nearly six months. The benefits of his family's self-care and health care became evident to him as a result of this crisis.

He became a convert, moving from a crisis-motivated junkie to a self-care, health care, and quality-of-life motivated man. What a difference Lifestyle Care made in his life, and what a difference it will make in yours.

Health care is about keeping your body healthy and strong. Your body is designed to be healthy. Disease is not a normal part of everyday life. When it happens it is unfortunate, but we need to stop thinking of sickness as natural. This is like assuming that debt and bankruptcy are normal. They are not. Now, they can happen. And if they do, it's nice to know there is a Crisis Care system in place to get us back on track. But having to treat a disease is something we would all like to avoid if we can, and for most of us, we can.

Excellent health care, combined with great self-care, keeps your entire body functioning at its optimum level. While we all brush our teeth and floss after each meal (don't we?), we still see our dentist at least once or twice a year for a thorough examination. Dentistry was the first profession that packaged self-care, health care, and Crisis Care so that it made sense to the consumer. Most people clearly understand the value of keeping your teeth healthy, clean, and white while avoiding the dreaded root canal.

Chiropractors have also done a terrific job packaging the Health Care Hierarchy for the spine and nervous system. Just like nobody wants a root canal, people would prefer to keep their spine and nervous system healthy, balanced, and aligned throughout their lifetime. They want to be able to stay active as they age. We've all seen an elderly person whose spine is bent over and crooked from years of neglect and said to ourselves, "I don't want to end up like that." These crippled people didn't just wake up like that one day. Their spine grew wrong over time as their nerves deteriorated over time. Haven't you also seen the unfortunate soul who neglected his or her spine and ended up with a herniated or ruptured disk? Ouch. It only takes one bad disk to put a damper on your quality of life as you age. Given the relationship between the spine and nervous system and all of the ill effects that come with preventable spinal problems, no wonder millions of people swear by their chiropractic care and have made it such an important part of their 100 Year Lifestyle.

THE IMPORTANCE OF EARLY DETECTION

Our current medical system is not really health care at all. It is almost all about Crisis Care. The emphasis on early detection, however, is an important aspect of health care because research has shown that if you are inflicted with a serious illness, early detection increases your chances of full recovery. Early detection won't get you in the best shape of your life or help you avoid the crisis. If it's been detected, you are in crisis. If you know of diseases in your family history, make the lifestyle changes we've discussed. Your likelihood of contracting these conditions could decrease substantially. Prioritize the known conditions in your family history when scheduling early detection screenings. For example, if heart disease runs in your family, make early detection examinations with a cardiologist. Your physician will monitor your heart to help you with early detection. If you are at risk, a good doctor will first talk to you about lifestyle changes you need to make. This may mean leaner meats, more fruits and vegetables, and less sodium – exactly what we've already discussed. However, if you find that these recommendations are fairly limited, consult a nutritionist. Physicians study very little about nutrition in medical school and are more inclined to recommend drugs. Do your homework and look to change your life before making medication your life. The long term side effects of these drugs can severely affect your health.

If colon cancer is a part of your history, make the lifestyle changes we've discussed and follow the recommended schedule for colon screenings.

One major problem with medical screenings is that they can often give you false positives. If you get a positive test, you might want to redo the test a second or third time before you panic. False positives are very common. Also, always consider getting second opinions on any course of action, as you would be amazed how opinions can vary from one provider to the next. We found this to be true firsthand when my wife, Lisa, was pregnant with our oldest son, Jacob. Her blood sugar was slightly elevated and her initial obstetrician recommended radical and aggressive procedures to monitor her blood sugar. We did not agree with his recommendations. Our personal research and gut feeling told us that this was unnecessary, and we went on a search for a second and third opinion. We found that the differences between obstetricians were massive. Finally we came upon a doctor who we felt was right on in his recommendations. We monitored her blood sugar through nutrition and exercise, she received chiropractic adjustments weekly and Jacob was born a healthy baby. We avoided an intensely aggressive protocol with a much higher risk of side effects for both Mommy and Baby.

PREVENTION

Many people confuse early detection with prevention. There is a big difference. Early detection consists of engaging in diagnostic testing for the purpose of identifying a condition in its earliest stages. This is not the same as prevention, which is what a healthy 100 Year Lifestyle can help you achieve. Millions of people have a chiropractor and nutritionist as their health care specialists and their medical physician as their disease specialist.

One interesting side note is important as I write this section. I can hear the voices on the extremes of the antimedical side screaming about all of the medical mishaps that happen and saying that they would never go to a medical doctor. Based on the statistics that reveal medical errors as a leading cause of death, their concern has merit. Interestingly, I have seen dozens of these people end up in the hospital and under the knife, having their lives saved by a dedicated medical professional. Afterward, they often ease their position as they see how their role is important when placed in the proper place in the Health Care Hierarchy.

I have also heard the voices of old-time medical physicians who for decades badmouthed the chiropractic profession and other up-and-coming health care providers, such as acupuncturists, massage therapists, personal trainers, nutritionists, and others. Now, many of them are utilizing their services regularly to stay healthy. In my practice I saw dozens of medical physicians and their families who were committed to chiropractic Lifestyle Care, and I know many of my colleagues who do the same. There is an important place for everyone and at some time or another we may want and need all of these professionals in our lives.

HEALTH CARE PROVIDERS AND THE LIFESTYLE CARE CONTINUUM

There are many health care providers that you can see to help you reach your health goals. This includes your chiropractor to keep your spine and nervous system healthy, nutritionists to keep your diet healthy, personal trainers to personalize your fitness program, and your dentist to keep your teeth clean. True health care providers work with you on expressing your Innate health potential and keeping you at the top of your game. They promote your optimum health and well-being.

The Lifestyle Care Continuum defines the ways that you can participate with your health care providers. The first way is Crisis Care. The goal of Crisis Care is to give you relief from your current condition and bring stability to your body. The Critical Transition is continuing with your care and lifestyle changes, whether you are experiencing symptoms or not, so that your body can regenerate and heal itself for the long term. Lifestyle Care will keep you healthy and functioning at your highest level. To learn more, visit www.100yearlifestyle.com and click on Health Care Philosophy."

Dentists, like Dr. Debra King from the Atlanta Center for Cosmetic Dentistry, not only help keep your teeth and gums healthy, but they also keep the rest of your body healthy as well. Studies have revealed that good oral health is a factor in maintaining your overall well-being.

Dr. King has been a personal friend and my family's dentist for the last 25 years. I have watched her practice grow and thrive by applying the principles of The 100 Year Lifestyle. Her staff is exceptional at Crisis Care handling everything including cracked teeth, cavities and crowns. They do fantastic work with Lifestyle Care by providing a range of services to keep your smile clean, bright, and white for a lifetime and their highly trained team of doctors and hygienists are very committed to educating people through the Critical Transition from Crisis Care to Lifestyle Care. Their commitment to these principles has made the Atlanta Center for Cosmetic Dentistry one of the premiere dental offices in the world.

Optometrists help to maintain eye health. They diagnose eye problems and vision disease, prescribe eyeglasses, and can even help you strengthen your eyes with exercises. Podiatrists provide foot care that is important to your feet, which can affect the structure of your entire body. Orthotics and foot supports, especially ones that are custom designed to your feet, are something that all active people should consider and can be obtained at a variety of places including chiropractic offices, podiatric offices and shoe stores that sell custom-made shoes, since foot alignment can also effect spinal alignment.

CHIROPRACTIC CARE

Chiropractic care is a vital health care option that every person should utilize throughout their lifetime. It was founded on the principles that are readily accepted by all health care providers today, that human beings have within them an Innate Intelligence that is self-healing and self-regulating. The body has the ability to stay healthy as long as there is no interference. Initially chiropractors attracted patients who were the sickest of the sick and many of these patients healed miraculously.

While many conditions are helped through chiropractic care, the purpose of the care is not to treat symptoms but to align the spine and remove interference from the nervous system so the body can heal itself and restore itself to normal function. Research has shown conclusively, that when pressure is placed on spinal nerves the body breaks down and when the pressure is removed the body begins to heal. This is why healthy people as well as sick people are attracted to chiropractic care—both as an important part of their Crisis Care as well as for Lifestyle Care.

Many professional athletes and sports teams utilize chiropractic care to recover quickly from injuries and maximize their athletic performance. You hear people all the time say about chiropractic care, "I don't know how people live without it!" Occasionally you will hear the Crisis Care skeptic say that once you begin chiropractic care you will have to go for the rest of your life. This is not true. There is no "have to." If you want to stay healthy, you will find that the intensity of your Lifestyle Care will depend on the intensity of your lifestyle. It's like going to the dentist. The more you brush and floss and the less sugar you consume, the less frequent and intense your dental visits will be.

The frequency and intensity of the care you'll require will depend on the amount of self-care you give your spine on a daily basis. Good self-care habits including having good posture, practicing yoga, and doing stretches, as well as good sleeping, sitting, and stress management habits will ensure that your spine and nervous system stay healthy. Your Lifestyle Care will be less frequent. The more you neglect your self-care, the more frequently you will need to be adjusted.

The Benefits of Lifestyle Care

The benefits of Lifestyle Care are many and well documented. From improving athletic performance, increasing brain function and increasing bone density to strengthening the immune system and preventing deterioration, the results can be dramatic. And as common sense and world renowned 100 Year Lifestyle Affiliate chiropractor, Dr. Ernie Landi has stated so eloquently, "If you prevent it, you don't have to treat it."

Lifestyle Care is about keeping your spine and nervous system aligned, balanced and functioning to its full potential throughout your lifetime. This allows your brain and your body to communicate efficiently without interference so that they can function at their highest level and help you enjoy life to the fullest.

People will frequently ask, "This makes a lot of sense. How often should I get my spine and nervous system checked?" The answer is quite simple and depends a lot on you. The intensity of your Lifestyle Care will depend on the intensity of your lifestyle as well as the underlying condition of your spine and nervous system. People who live stress free lives and have no underlying deterioration require much less Lifestyle Care.

On the other hand, people with moderate amounts of stress and deterioration require more frequent visits and people who are under severe stress or have a lot of deterioration require much more frequent visits to keep their body functioning at high levels of health. You and your chiropractor will determine together the frequency that is best for you based on your personal health condition and goals.

As the intensity of your lifestyle changes from month to month or from year to year you may find that the intensity of your Lifestyle Care also needs to change. For example, if you have found that an adjustment every two weeks has been ideal for you, then you change to a more stressful job with a lot of sitting or a long commute, you and your chiropractor may find that a weekly adjustment works better.

If you are a casual exerciser and decide to start participating in triathlons, the increased intensity of your training might require you to increase the intensity of your visits to multiple times per week. On the other hand, if your life becomes less stressful, you begin meditating three times a day and your underlying spinal conditions have already been corrected, you may find that your Lifestyle Care frequency may decrease in its intensity.

The most important thing for you to understand is that Lifestyle Care is not based on symptoms. Your frequency is not determined by how you feel but instead is determined by whether or not you have a subluxation, a spinal imbalance with nerve pressure, that needs to be adjusted. Since additional research has revealed that nerve compression can exist without pain, waiting until you have symptoms to get checked is not a good idea. Only your chiropractor can determine whether you need an adjustment or not through a chiropractic check-up.

Ask around and you will find that there are millions of people who have been under chiropractic care for decades not just because they have had a problem but because they have experienced the benefits of Lifestyle Care. These people may be some of the healthiest people you meet. Too many people in our society are suffering because they are crisis oriented when it comes to their health. Don't let this happen to you. It is easier, less expensive and more fun to stay well than it is to have to get well after you become sick or injured. People who live The 100 Year Lifestyle take the lessons from the nursing home generation seriously and make this shift from Crisis Care to Lifestyle Care.

Fortunately, chiropractic has grown up over the past 118 years and there are now many types of chiropractic procedures and techniques—from the traditional adjustment where you here the "sound" of the spine being adjusted to very light touch, soft-tissue techniques by hand or through the use of computer technology and instruments that balance the spine. Some techniques work better for some people than others, but the important thing is to find the one that works best for you and to utilize that care as a part of your lifestyle. The best news of all is that chiropractic is one of the safest forms of health care, with extremely low incidences of malpractice and patient injury. Aside from the occasional scare campaign by special interest dinosaur groups, chiropractors work very well with all types of physicians to do what is in the best interest of their patients.

You can find The 100 Year Lifestyle Affiliate Chiropractor near you at www.100yearlifestyle.com.

No Sick Days for This Kid – Morgan Handt, DC

As a kid growing up in a chiropractic family, I was very different than many of my friends. For starters, my brothers and I were never vaccinated, and we never took medications for anything. No Tylenol, Advil, cough syrup or allergy medications would ever be found in our home. My parents always told us that the power that made out bodies would heal our bodies, and those are the words that we live by. We received chiropractic checkups from the moment that we were born so that our bodies would work the way they were intended to, perfectly.

I remember when I was little that my friends would always be absent from class on random days throughout the year because they were sick, and I didn't understand why they were so lucky, missing school all the time when I was always there. After hearing this over and over, my mom decided that if I wanted a day off from school, and I had no tests, that I could ask her for one. Since I never got sick, I got to have fun on my "sick days". Now I was the luckiest kid in school! Later on she told me that what she was giving me were mental health days, and I understood very clearly what she meant.

When I became an adult, I became much more aware of how different my lifestyle was, and how healthy I was. I decided to follow in my father's footsteps and became a chiropractor. It is such a great feeling to know that I am helping families of this generation to have healthy happy lives, expressing their full potential for a lifetime.

ESSENTIAL INNERVATION – YOUR BODY'S NATURAL I.T. SYSTEM

In today's virtual world we all know the importance of a healthy I.T. system. This Information and Technology (I.T.) infrastructure is necessary for our homes, offices, and the communication between our loved ones to function properly. Wired and wireless, we count on this I.T. system every minute of every day. Within you, your Nervous System acts as your natural I.T. system to keep your body functioning properly by supplying your cells with Innervation.

Innervation is defined as the "distribution of nerve fibers to an organ or body region." Innervation is essential for the health of every cell, tissue and organ of your body. More than 45 miles of nerves connect your brain to your skin alone. Innervation between your brain and your heart, lungs, liver, kidneys, and muscles relays up to three million messages every second. This Essential Innervation monitors both your inner and outer world and adapts you to your environment. With the right training, your I.T. system can even help you execute the perfect golf swing or climb a mountain. Unfortunately, our tendency is to neglect our internal I.T. system until it breaks down. This is not a healthy choice!

When it comes to your health, healing, or optimizing your health potential, there are some important things that you must know about it.

Life is not possible without this Essential Innervation. In his book Healing and the Mind, Bill Moyers found that immune system cells stop working when innervation is removed. We have all heard stories of people who have suffered brain or spinal cord injuries whose lives were cut short or whose bodies completely stopped functioning because they were paralyzed. Researchers are working tirelessly to find solutions to replace it when it is lost. Your natural I.T. system should not be taken for granted, ever.

When Innervation is interfered with by vertebral subluxation, or other injuries, only partial function is possible. Research out of the University of Colorado found that pressure on the nerve equivalent to the weight of a dime can reduce nerve transmission. Stretching a nerve by 6 percent can decrease the strength of its impulse by 70 percent. Interference to your I.T. system can cause immediate symptoms from colic in a baby to allergies, breathing difficulties, headaches or any type of pain. Because of the vast nature of the nervous system, the symptoms can mimic many diagnoses, even unexplainable ones. This is one reason why people with a myriad of symptoms get results with chiropractic care. Because the focus is on removing the interference to it rather than just making a localized pain or condition feel better, the body can begin to heal itself right away.

Your body can function normally with proper Innervation. Every cell, tissue and organ can interact in a healthy way with accurate signals and messages being sent and received. Your ability to adapt to stress, digest food, eliminate waste, and perform daily tasks becomes second nature. With it, you may even be able to walk and chew gum at the same time since it works without you even thinking about it.

When you optimize it, you can achieve optimum health and peak performance levels and push your body to its limits. We see this in top performers and athletes, and every day people like you who run marathons or participate in Iron Man, Tough Mudder or other extreme activities. Lifestyle Care can help you optimize it, which is why most professional sports teams and athletes utilize chiropractic care in this way.

If you have not done so in the past 3 months, now is the time to evaluate the health of your natural I.T. system with a chiropractic examination. Innervation is essential to life, healing, health and vitality. Make the health of your natural I.T. system your top priority.

Essential Innervation – Your Body's Natural I.T. System
- Without IT, life is not possible
- If there is interference to IT, health is not possible
- With IT, health is your natural state
- Optimize IT and express your full potential

PERSONAL TRAINERS

The personal-training industry has become a field of specialists. If you are an athlete who is striving for peak performance, there are trainers who specialize in that. If you are looking to decrease your body fat to the normal range—12 to 15 percent for men and 15 to 20 percent for women— there are trainers who can help you with that. If you want to improve your cardiovascular fitness, you can also find trainers who specialize in that. The key to having success with your personal trainer is to clearly communicate your goals.

When you choose a personal trainer, make sure you find one that is certified. There are several professional associations that certify personal trainers and ensure that they are trained properly. Review your exercise program with your trainer every three to six months. Revisit your goals regularly as well, and maintain great communication with your trainer.

The Top 5 Traits of Successful Exercisers
by Mike Epstein, CPT, VP of Gold's Gym, Paramus, New Jersey, Board of Directors Gold's Gym International

1.   Successful exercisers are motivated.
2.   Successful exercisers educate themselves and seek professional assistance.
3.   Successful exercisers set small, obtainable and realistic goals.
4.   Successful exercisers make fitness a part of their lifestyle.
5.   Successful exercisers use visual feedback to measure their progress.

MASSAGE THERAPISTS

More and more people are utilizing massage therapists as a part of their health care team. Their level of training and standards of excellence have grown dramatically. Massage Therapy schools are popping up all over the country and post-graduate programs such as One Concept are bringing massage therapists together with other health care providers, including chiropractors, to promote an interconnected relationship that helps people achieve optimum health.

Massage has also been proven to relieve a variety of conditions such as many of the discomforts of pregnancy, like backaches, leg cramps, morning sickness, varicose veins, and headaches. Massage may even be used during labor to ease the pain and potentially shorten the labor. Some studies suggest that massage may also be an effective way to treat PMS. Massage can help your body heal from injuries as well. One in five Americans took advantage of massage last year; however, Crisis Care is only one way to utilize massage. Getting regular massage keeps your body stress free, relaxes you, and can keep you as healthy as possible. Determine the frequency that works best for you and make massage a part of your lifestyle.

NUTRITIONISTS AND DIETITIANS

Good nutrition is another key to good health care. "You are what you eat" is a true statement, since your breakfast in the morning will become a part of your body by the afternoon. Keep yourself healthy with good nutrition. A certified dietitian or nutritionist can help you develop an eating plan that fits your lifestyle and your current health condition. They can also help you choose a supplement program that can fill in the gaps of your diet and give you extra support to counterbalance your family history.

Supplementation is important in today's world since most of us don't always eat properly and can be challenged by excess stress.

Take advantage of the health care resources in your community and the odds will be in your favor that you will prevent and avoid a crisis while enjoying optimum health and peak performance levels throughout your lifetime.

Centenarian Secret
Learn to love the things that are good for you. ☺

CHAPTER 10

CRISIS CARE: PREPARING FOR AND AVOIDING A CRISIS-FILLED LIFE

At some time or another we will all have a crisis. Being Prepared will ensure that our minds and bodies recover as quickly as possible and our pocketbooks recover quickly as well. Having a Crisis Care team of health care specialists you can trust is certainly important in times of need. You will develop this Crisis Care team as you explore and practice the self-care and health care elements of the Health Care Hierarchy because you will be surrounding yourself with trusted experts and voices. This is important.

Our current system is both bankrupt and broken. The system is supposed to make things better and always do right by us. That doesn't always happen and we are bitterly disappointed when it doesn't. On top of that, people all too often feel dehumanized in the process—regarded as mere numbers rather than human beings. You absolutely need to research health insurance policies and find one that fits you and your family. It is important to have crisis coverage in place. This is why a good insurance agent can be such an important part of your health care team and why you should review your policies regularly, as they can become outdated as your needs change with age. You must be your own advocate for the best care as well as the best options for financing your care.

The High Cost of Crisis Care

Crisis Care is bankrupting our country and causing tremendous unnecessary suffering to individuals and families. As an example, look at the following numbers:

Condition	Cost per Year
Back Pain	$86 Billion
Cancer	$228 Billion
Heart Disease	$316 Billion
Diabetes	$174 Billion
Obesity	$147 Billion

The total cost for just these five conditions is $951 Billion which is the equivalent of $3,100.00 per every man, woman and child per year whether you have this condition or not. Keep in mind that this does not include every other diagnosed condition that we did not mention including allergies, ulcers, thyroid conditions, intestinal disorders, etc.

If you and your family have suffered some type of health crisis, then your numbers are substantially higher because of the direct effect that these conditions are having on your life and your family. The Crisis Care model of not taking care of yourself again until you have another crisis won't work for an extended life span. This attitude, a 60 year lifestyle, can lead to decades of unnecessary suffering.

On the other hand, the Health Care Hierarchy of The 100 Year Lifestyle puts self-care and health care first and Crisis Care last, hopefully avoiding crisis altogether.

Lifestyle Care is a much better option because of its preventative nature. When you look at the conditions listed above and do the research a majority of these conditions and expenses would never occur if we all took this proactive approach. Isn't it time that you and your loved ones break this cycle of crisis? What are you waiting for?

Health insurance as we know it today is really crisis insurance. If you get sick or injured, your policy, if you have one, will partially cover your costs. When I first got into practice, it was common for people to have $100 deductible policies with 90 percent coverage. This sure seems like an eternity ago. Contracts now limit coverage, cap costs, and incite doctors to not recommend certain treatments. Insurance companies and the government are trying to adapt to a changing marketplace, but if you or a loved one has had a crisis in the past decade or so, you are likely to have had some issues with your insurer. All of us have experienced rising costs and declining benefits. How many times have you changed insurance companies over the past 20 or so years? How many times have your policy premiums changed? Have your premiums gone up? Mine sure have. Have your benefits gone down? You're not alone—we are all in the same boat.

THE RIGHT APPROACH TO CRISIS CARE

Most importantly, accept responsibility for your own health care. You are ultimately responsible for your own health. This means staying informed and educating yourself, especially in times of a crisis. You want the best doctors and the best health care providers on your team.

When you consult with your doctor, be prepared. Do some background reading beforehand. Research online and look into your situation. Use the Internet, along with your inner guidance, to assist you in understanding your problem so that you can be a part of the solution.

> **Centenarian Secret**
> Think of your health insurance along the same lines as homeowner's insurance. You don't have homeowner's insurance to keep your carpets clean or wipe your counters. You are responsible for these things. You are covered in case of a crisis. Day to day, you must keep your home looking good and prevent it from deteriorating. Your health requires the same day-to-day upkeep from you.

Doctors are not gods; they are human beings just like you and me who happen to have an expertise in a given area. Every doctor or specialist you see might give you a different opinion, and there are numerous noninvasive options available today for you to explore. Many procedures, such as chiropractic, that were written off in the past by the political and financial powers are now mainstream and widely accepted.

Chiropractic has been a profession since 1895. Acupuncture is an ancient Chinese treatment that has been used in the United States for around 30 years.

So start by looking in a mirror. Turn and look at the health of your spine and nervous system. Are you standing up as straight as you once did, or are you starting to slouch? Whose responsibility is this? Is your heart growing healthier and stronger as time goes by? Or is it weaker? Your health is ultimately your responsibility—not your doctor's, and certainly not your insurance company's.

LIVE LONG AND STRONG EXERCISE
The proactive steps I should take to remain healthy and avoid a possible crisis are:
1. _____
2. _____
3. _____
4. _____
5. _____

Don't confuse Crisis Care with health care. For example, if every time you have the sniffles you take an antibiotic because you believe that antibiotics will help your sniffles, you are setting your immune system up for failure. Hospitals are filled with super bugs, or antibiotic resistant bacteria because of the overuse of these potentially dangerous drugs. They are prolonging patient stays, increasing medical fees, and even leading to thousands of unnecessary deaths—all because of the overuse of antibiotics. Be careful of biased science that sells a procedure. Do your homework and really learn to trust yourself.

OPTIONS

There are so many self-care and health care options out there today and the choices can be overwhelming. Where should you begin? Recently a very prominent member of the community where I live had an unexpected heart attack. It became a wake-up call for him and he made the commitment to change his life. His crisis was a motivator for him. It also became a quality-of-life motivator for hundreds of other people in the community. Every type of doctor in town—from the chiropractor to the cardiologist—ended up with bookings from this one incident. People had been putting off their vital health care. Gym memberships increased too, and heart-rate-monitor sales took a leap. Don't wait for a crisis to motivate you. Choose quality of life motivation instead, and make it your lifestyle.

Trust yourself. With everything we have discussed so far, where do you think you should begin? Do you have someone in your life whose health you would like to model? Ask for a recommendation of their providers. Interview a chiropractor, a general practitioner, or a cardiologist. Attend a lecture, listen to an audio, and educate yourself. Begin your discussions with a personal trainer or a nutritionist. Look into a new bed or a safer chair. Start shopping around and make a commitment that gets you in the self-care, health care game.

At some point in your life you are going to make this choice. I hope you make yours because you want to, and not because you were forced into it because of a crisis. Let's get our priorities straight so we can all enjoy The 100 Year Lifestyle we desire with the quality of life we deserve.

THE 100 YEAR LIFESTYLE
ACTION PLAN FOR LASTING CHANGE

1. Choose your own hierarchy. If your Health Care Hierarchy has been crisis motivated and you have been on a crisis roller coaster, choose to make self-care a priority, and get yourself on track. Decide which self-care strategies are the most appealing to you and begin to make them a part of your lifestyle, one day at a time, and one choice at a time.

2. Remember Life Changing Principle Number 1: Change is easy—thinking about change is hard. It's time to make the changes you know you need to make. Stop thinking and take your first action step. Go for a walk, join a gym, and set an appointment with a personal trainer, a chiropractor, or a cardiologist. Pick up the phone now and make the call. Don't put it off.

3. Trust yourself. You know what you need to do first. Trust yourself and follow your instincts. Get on the path and stay on your path with Life Changing Principle Number 2, and make every choice count.

4. Educate yourself. Become an expert in your ideal 100 Year Lifestyle by reading about all of the things that matter to your health so that you can become well informed and support yourself in achieving your goals. You will also be better equipped to handle any crisis that might occur if you have prepared yourself through this educational process.

5. Build a team. Build your ideal self-care, health care and Crisis Care team. You probably have many of these relationships already established, and there may be some that you need to add. Do your homework. Ask your family, friends, and neighbors about their "team members" and make the appropriate appointments. Meet your team and begin implementing the game plan that you know will make a difference for you.

6. Enjoy the journey. This educational process can be fun and exciting. Your mind will begin to feel younger and your body will also, with each commitment you make.

7. Bring a friend along for the ride. Nobody wants to be alone while traveling this path. Share this process with others now so that you can enjoy the journey together for 100 years and beyond.

PART 5

Creating the Ideal Environment You Can Enjoy for 100 Years

It's about the journey.
Immerse yourself!

CHAPTER 11

ENJOY YOUR ENVIRONMENT AND MAKE THE MOST OF YOUR JOURNEY

If you are going to live an active, healthy quality of life to 100, your environment will play a key role in how much you enjoy the journey. So go ahead, immerse yourself!

LASTING CHANGE REQUIRES CHANGING YOUR ENVIRONMENT.

The truth is that The 100 Year Lifestyle is not just about getting to 100 at all. It's not just about running a marathon to 100 and then collapsing at the finish line. It is actually more about the journey. It is not just about a quantity of years. It is about the quality of the quantity of years that you live, so that whether you make it to 80, 90, 100, or 110, you make the most of every day along the way. The environments you create—both the internal environment within your mind and body and the external environment where you live, work, and play—will have a lot to do with how much you enjoy your journey.

> **Centenarian Secret**
> Here is an important question to ask yourself that is a key to you making the most of your 100 Year Lifestyle. How much fun are you having?

Close your eyes after you finish this paragraph and perform this visualization with me. Describe and visualize your ideal environment. Begin with yourself: your ideal health, energy, and shape. Visualize the inner peace and personal confidence that you want. Picture yourself using your creativity and talents. Imagine using those talents to achieve mastery over something that you enjoy and can sustain you—for the rest of your life. Maybe you have a love of words and communication. Imagine using that skill to help others through writing, speaking or teaching. Or maybe you "communicate" with your hands or are creative—you love to paint or draw. Imagine drawing on and cultivating those talents as a part of your lifestyle. Maybe you are a healer or an excellent problem solver? Are you utilizing these gifts to your capabilities? You will find the greatest fulfillment when you connect with and then act on your Innate talents throughout your life. So imagine the rest of your 100 years with this in mind. Close your eyes for a moment now and visualize your ideal environment.

Now describe your ideal external environment. Really get into the visualization so you can experience it with all of your senses. See the colors of your ideal environment, your home, your car, your office, and your vacations. What are the things that you would be doing to enjoy each day to the fullest? What are some outrageous goals you would like to achieve? Is your environment filled with trees, an ocean, lake, or river? Does it include the mountains? Are you passionate about your work? What type of people are you surrounded with? How much fun are you having and what is making life fun?

Now that you've gone through this experience and you have opened your eyes, answer this question: Are you living your ideal 100 Year Lifestyle? Is your current environment one that you can enjoy for the balance of your years? Is it a good starting point? If yes, what a fabulous foundation you have to build on. If not, get excited about the transition from where you are to where you want to be, and get ready to enjoy the journey.

There are three aspects of your environment that are important to consider in relation to creating your ideal 100 Year Lifestyle:

1. **Your inner environment.** Create a compelling vision for the rest of your life that is aligned with your Innate Intelligence and develop the mindset, focus and health to make it happen. It's got to come from within you.

2. **Your external environment.** Live, work, and play in the ideal external environment that resonates with your Innate Intelligence. Once you have the clarity, you can create and manifest your ideal environment. Sometimes this will happen quickly and sometimes slowly. The key is to move in the right direction, toward what you really want, one choice at a time. This will align your internal and external environments. Also, place yourself in external environments that feed your internal creativity. This will help you to attract, live and build your ideal 100 Year Lifestyle with ease.

3. **Congruency between your internal and external environments.** Congruence between your words and your actions is powerful. Many people call it walking the talk. People who walk the talk have an inner strength regardless of their size, physical attributes, or age. Their integrity shines through. They have a presence about them that is appealing and attractive. The greater the level of congruency between your internal and external environments, the more magnetic you will be at attracting what you want.

The relationship between your internal environment and your external environment is crucial to a healthy, passionate, prosperous life.

Your internal environment is the one between your two ears, and the one within your skin. It is your mind, body, and spirit. You are going to be the one that has to develop the vision for your life. If someone else does it for you, you will be living somebody else's 100 Year Lifestyle and not your own. The stress of this will cause an implosion and can eventually lead to all types of health problems, frustrations and challenges.

I remember hearing a speaker at a recent seminar talking about health and wellness. This particular speaker, while passionate and intense in his presentation and delivery, was 50 pounds overweight and looked stressed out of his mind. At the beginning of his presentation, the room was full. The topic was compelling. The message in the paragraph immediately following the title of his talk was very well written and designed to attract a lot of listeners—and it did.

As the speaker began to rant and rave, people began to slowly leave the room. By the end of the talk, there were only about half of the people left. The incongruence between his words and his "being" spoke volumes to the audience and drove them away, even though his message was compelling. This is the effect of incongruence in a speaker setting, and this is also the effect of incongruence in life.

I have seen incongruence between a person's internal and external environments cause frustration to them in so many ways, costing them money, love, and health. A few years ago I went to visit a chiropractor who wanted his practice to be filled with generations of kids and families for Lifestyle Care. He was an excellent doctor and had taken a lot of extra training necessary to develop his skills in this area. He wanted to be a community leader for health and longevity.

This doctor had the financial backing of his parents, who wanted him to have the nicest office on the planet. They put him through school, found his location, and built out one of the most beautiful offices I have ever seen. It was a great external environment.

Unfortunately for this excellent doctor, they also decorated the office like his grandmother's living room. You know what I mean, the kind where everything is so perfect that you are afraid to leave a footprint on the carpet, a fingerprint on the counter, or a butt print on the couch. No matter how hard this doctor tried to attract families to his practice for care, he couldn't do it. People were afraid they would mess up his beautiful space. It was not the ideal environment for families, even though in his heart, that is what he wanted to attract. This incongruence cost him dearly until he finally changed his environment.

At first he resisted these changes that I knew he needed to make. He argued for why he couldn't make the changes. Eventually, he recognized the reality of his situation and the need to make some external changes that were more congruent with his internal vision for his practice. He immediately became more magnetic, attracting more of the types of people that he wanted to see in his practice.

He became a 100 Year Lifestyle Affiliate office and changed his environment. He changed the coffee table from sharp, pointy edge glass to rounded corners. He put some fresh, educational posters and immersed his practice in new, up to date educational resources. He changed his website to match his internal message and standard of care. These changes were subtle but huge because they created a congruency with his internal environment, and he turned his practice around overnight. The message was clear and his patients found it easy to get The Big Idea.

Now is the time to upgrade your environments and fully enjoy the journey every step of the way.

CHAPTER 12

CREATING YOUR IDEAL INTERNAL ENVIRONMENT WHEREVER YOU GO

We have already spent quite a bit of time on your internal environment. We've worked a lot on getting your mindset excited about the opportunities that come with an extended life span and have given you strategies to maintain youthful energy. We've shown you how to eliminate destructive patterns that are taking years off your life and helped you establish the health habits of Lifestyle Care.

Now it's time to create the vision for your extended life so that the rest of your life is exciting, inspiring, and one that you want to live, remembering Life Changing Principle Number 3: Approach Change with Your Ideal 100 Year Lifestyle in mind. The fact is that if you do not have a vision for your life with exciting new goals to achieve and things to accomplish, then you are going to have to create it. The more clearly you can visualize it, the more likely you will be able to transition to it immediately and over time, and the more fun the rest of your life will be. What is your ideal lifestyle? The one you would like to live? If you do not develop a clear vision to construct your future, you will end up reconstructing your past over and over again.

One of the challenges of today's centenarians has been a lack of vision for their later years. Once they retire they spend their days watching the news and checking the mail. This gets old quickly and makes you old quickly too. There are so many exciting options when you continue to set new goals, challenge yourself, and explore your inner and outer world. It's your decision, and you are the one who is going to have to make it happen.

Centenarian Secret
You can either construct your future, or you can continue to reconstruct the past. But you can't do both at the same time. You have to choose.

There is an old saying in the consulting world that goes something like this: Take a successful business owner and put him or her in a failing business and they will turn that business around and make it successful. On the other hand, if you take the owner of a failing business and put him or her in a successful one, it won't be too long before they turn that business around, and drive it into the ground. I have seen many doctors do this to their practices. I have seen numerous people do this in their lives. They move into a new town and they unconsciously re-create their life exactly as it was in the previous location. You are at the perfect starting place to set up things exactly as you want if you are willing to change your mind and create a compelling vision for your future.

And as you transition yourself with Life Changing Principle Number 2, make sure you acknowledge your progress along the way because changing your environment is a process that takes time—unless you were like me and were forced there by a crisis.

This happened to me in 1994, a time when I wanted to make a lot of changes in my life. I was in my early thirties; I had a young family, a growing practice, and was working only 20 miles from home, but the commuter traffic kept me in the car much more than I wanted.

The strain of trying to make everything fit together was affecting my work life and my family life. I wanted to move my office closer to home; however, my office was in a great location—on Peachtree Road in Buckhead, which is an affluent and very commercial part of Atlanta. I was reluctant to make the change. I had a terrific practice and I was established there. Fear of the unknown kept me stuck in place. I didn't know if my practice members would follow me to a new location or if I could build an equally successful practice in another part of town. I also knew that I wanted to change the environment of that office. It had become stifling because my practice had grown so much that the original layout of the office had created capacity issues and flow problems as we grew. People had to wait for a longer period of time than they really should have, and all of this was due to the structure of the environment.

I stayed stuck for a while. Eventually it took a crisis for me to make the changes I knew I needed to make. The crisis came in the form of a little old lady who lost control of her car in the parking lot, stepped on the gas instead of the brakes, and ploughed her car right through the center of my office at 40 miles per hour. Can you imagine that? I had the first drive-through chiropractic office in history. Thank God this happened just before my busiest time with patients, so there were only a few people in the office. Initially I was really traumatized. I wasn't thinking clearly, I didn't know what to do, and I was having some post-traumatic stress. My internal environment was not functioning in a healthy way. All I could see was the destruction in my external environment. It was like I had blinders on that blocked out the possibilities that existed from the destruction.

Around a week later, with the help of my wife and some good friends and family members, I realized that I needed to start thinking about the situation differently. Yes, I had this destruction happening that needed to be cleaned up. Yes, I had this challenge and I knew internally that I could either continue to play the victim, or I could shift my environment. There were so many changes that I had been wanting to make to the layout of the office so it would flow better. Finally, I decided to view the crisis as an opportunity to make the changes that I had wanted to make for a long time. I began to look for the good and seek out the opportunities that were delivered by this angel. What happened then was miraculous.

I started to get excited about the opportunity to re-create my vision. I realized now, because of the accident, I could do it and save the demolition costs. It was an opportunity to set up the office to help more people. Also, I decided that maybe this was the time to move and open a second office. I began to drive around my home neighborhood and see if there were any new office locations that were available. The ideal space that I had been looking at within a mile of my house became available that day. I got psyched, and within two months, I opened a second office right where I wanted to be. The opportunity was right there but I wouldn't have seen it if I wasn't willing to change my mind about the situation and open up to acting on my vision and building a compelling future. I learned to package my thoughts differently. I learned to turn the crisis into an opportunity.

GET CREATIVE AND USE SOME DIFFERENT LOBULES OF YOUR BRAIN

The opportunity that we all have because of potential longevity is incredible. We have the chance to learn—and to use what we learn over time to continue to build our lives. What a great gift it is to be able to break out of old patterns that keep us trapped. This is what I call "a lobule jump," referring to the different parts of the brain (called *lobules*) we use to perform certain tasks and solve problems. Rather than getting caught up in a certain thought pattern, which can lead to overanalyzing and paralysis of analysis, you can open up your mind to see things differently by shifting to a different lobule of your brain.

Very often we get stuck seeing things a certain way rather than using our entire mind to see all sides. Like a holograph that changes pictures when you change your angle, so does nearly every situation that relates to your environment—you've just got to be willing to stretch your brain to see things differently.

When was the last time you looked at a picture of a brain? Isn't it amazing that this mass of matter, when animated with life, can run your entire body, adapt you to your environment, and originate thought? In computer scans you can see these lobules light up when they process information. For instance, the right lobule may activate when the brain is reading or interpreting language and the left side when you are translating complex mathematics or conducting three-dimensional visualization.

In fact, researchers performing postmortem studies on the brain of Albert Einstein found that his left inferior parietal lobule was larger than in most humans. The study, published in the *Lancet* in 1999, postulated that both Einstein's left lobule (the one responsible for complex mathematic calculations and spatial reasoning) and the right lobule might have expanded early in his prenatal development. You can make a lobule jump by asking yourself different questions and taking new actions based on the new answers.

I remember working with a patient who was having a lot of trouble with her spine and nervous system. She was severely subluxated. She was in a really stressful job and was sitting at work for about ten hours a day. She would then go home and wouldn't eat properly or exercise, and just crash on the couch and sit there until bedtime. She loved her chiropractic care because she always felt better, more aligned and balanced when she got adjusted, but she would continually re-create her problems by the way she was living her life.

Every other aspect of her environment—from the way she thought, sat, and ate, to the way she structured her day was destructive. I spoke with her about changing her internal environment—from the way she thought to the way she ate to the way she exercised. On top of that, I also advised her on ways to change her external environment—from where she ate to where she shopped to how she spent her day.

Changing her environment, both internal and external, was important for producing lasting change to her quality of life. It was amazing because by making these changes, she was able to end the destructive patterns that held her back. She was able to take her health to the next level, and this began to spill over into the rest of her life.

Centenarian Secret
Create a compelling vision for the rest of your life. What do you want to accomplish? What goals do you want to achieve? What experiences would you like to explore?

Don't get stuck operating in only one part of your brain when approaching challenges and opportunities. Make a lobule jump to move past negative self-perceptions or disempowering thoughts. By staying in the same part of the brain instead of expanding into other lobules, you may create the same scenarios over and over again.

Lobule jumping is a metaphor for opening up to new opportunities and possibilities and moving past mental obstacles. If you keep doing the same thing you always do, you're going to keep getting the same thing you always get. The easiest way to make a lobule jump is to simply start asking different questions of yourself, listening to your answers, and taking action. That may simply mean accepting the situation at first, and then taking the appropriate action steps that move you in the direction of your new life.

What does this look like to you? I think of my wife's grandfather, Hyman Sperling, who lived over 100 years. He was a special man and very dear to our family. In 1992, he lost his house during a hurricane. He was in his mid-eighties and had to rebuild his life from scratch. I asked him about it and his response came from a place of wisdom and certainty. "What is there to talk about?" he said. "It was a hurricane; it destroyed the house, the furniture, and everything in it. All we salvaged were some clothes. That's all." There was no pity, no analysis—although, maybe a touch of anger. The key was that he took action. "So we moved and started over. There was an apartment available in Coral Springs. We took it. I think it was $700 a month and we had to pay a three-month advance. We lived there for six weeks until we got out of there and bought an apartment in Palm Springs."

Change is easy. Thinking about change is hard. In times of crisis, always think and apply the Life Changing Principles of The 100 Year Lifestyle.

CHANGE THE WAY YOU THINK

You can change your life by changing the way you think. By using different pathways and asking new questions, you can connect to your Innate Intelligence and find exciting solutions.

LIVE LONG AND STRONG

Start lighting up new lobules of your brain to create a life without limits by asking these core questions:

- How can I be more effective in my life?
- What are the cores values that I want to base my life on?
- Who can be my mentor and help me achieve my goals?
- How can I be a better professional?
- What would make me a better listener?
- Who do I need to learn from to do my job better?
- How can I make myself heard in a positive way?
- What habit can I commit to that will change my life for the better?
- What commitments will make me a healthier person?
- What can I accept about my past that will enable me to move forward in my life?
- Who can I forgive today so that I can let go and live my life?
- What resources are available to me?
- What do I really want?
- Where do I want to live?
- What colors make me feel happy inside and would improve my environment?
- What changes can I make to my home to make it more enjoyable?
- What do I want my finances to be like in a year?
- What choices do I need to make to achieve that goal?
- What do I want from my life partner that I am not getting right now?
- How can I ask for it so that I am more likely to receive it?
- What do I need to give in order to have my partner feel secure?
- How can I use my talents and passions to earn extra money and make a difference?

Asking new and better questions will bring you answers that support your ideal 100 Year Lifestyle.

These types of questions open you up to greater possibilities that will invite exciting opportunities into your extended life. By acting on one or two of these at a time you will begin to attract the clarity that helps you create the environment you will enjoy for a lifetime. These are much better questions than … What are wrong with me? Why am I such an idiot? Why can't I reach my goals? Why bother, I am already 50 years old?

Negative thoughts can keep you in destructive patterns. Changing your thoughts about things can propel you into a human potential pattern that attracts your ideal 100 Year Lifestyle to you magnetically. Remember Life Changing Principle Number 1: Change is easy; thinking about change is hard. Dare yourself to dream and then make your dreams come true. After all, you get to start fresh with decades of experience under your belt. What an opportunity if you are willing to see it this way.

Think about the thoughts and attitudes you bring to every situation. Does the party get going when you get there or does it fall apart? Does a room feel more comfortable when you are there or do you create stress? Who ruins your day? Do you meet nice people wherever you go, or do you always find the jerk in the crowd? Do you find a financial opportunity in every situation? The one commonality in every environment you enter is you. You are going to take yourself with you wherever you go. Rather than judge yourself, you have an opportunity to look at the results you are creating and decide if you like them. If you don't like them, you can decide whether you want to change them—by changing your views and your vision. A change in your environment must begin with you.

Living The 100 Year Lifestyle: Neal and Lori Plasker

My cousin Neal is a good friend and an incredible man who just a few years ago lost his wife to cancer after a grueling 11-year battle. During that time he stood by her side with first-class integrity and commitment.

Initially when Barbara was diagnosed with lung cancer—a very rare form—the only hope for her was going to be a double lung transplant operation. They did all the necessary preparation and made arrangements to be on-call so Barbara could receive her new lungs. Finally the day came, and they flew to Birmingham for the surgery.

Lisa and I drove over to support them, as did several of our other family members. The surgery was a success. Barbara went through some intense rehabilitation and after several months was able to begin to enjoy her life again. She and Neal spent time with the kids and over the next few years, they got to see their youngest son get bar mitzvahed and their daughter get married, and attend several family members' high school and college graduations.

Ultimately, in August 2004, the cancer got the best of Barbara and the last few years of the battle were emotionally and physically exhausting for everyone in the family. Neal stood by Barbara's side and did his best to ease her suffering. His loyalty and commitment to her was a constant source of strength to the entire family.

Several months after Barbara's passing, Neal decided that he was still alive, and after many years of making the most of his life under difficult circumstances—which in my heart was a key to Barbara surviving so long—he decided he was ready to live life to the fullest, and he was open to finding love again. If there was anyone who deserved it, it was Neal. Several months later, he met a woman named Lori. They were a match.

Lori has her own story. She had a long but challenging marriage, which produced two beautiful children. Eventually, she found the courage to get a divorce. She continued to raise her daughters and got used to living on her own. Several years later, on her fiftieth birthday, she blew out the candles on her cake surrounded by close family and friends. Her life was full and good. She had completely healed from her divorce and she realized that she was deeply content and happy.

Soon afterward, a friend asked Lori about setting her up on a blind date. That man was Neal. Lori knew of Neal and had heard he was a good man. She remembers being very nervous on their first date. On their second date, Neal touched Lori's shoulder. Instantly Lori felt for the first time in a very long time that she was "home." Neal and Lori fell in love, got married, and are now building an incredible life together. They are doing a fabulous job blending their two families—Neal, with his three children, son-in-law, and new grandchild, and Lori, with her two daughters. They are committed to creating and sharing lots of great times and they have expanded their rock solid support system.

Neal and Lori have found true love after the age of 50 and got married. With a little luck and the principles of The 100 Year Lifestyle on his side, Neal and Lori could celebrate their silver, even a golden anniversary together, even though they are starting their journey together during midlife. Now with three grandchildren that they adore, they are certainly on their way.

ACCEPTING OUR CURRENT ENVIRONMENT

Dr. C is a chiropractor who, since implementing many of these 100 Year Lifestyle principles, has seen his patient base grow dramatically, his income has nearly tripled and he is having more fun than ever in his practice and his life. In the early stages of his training, he was an extremely stressed-out doctor. Every time one of his patients didn't do exactly what he wanted them to do, he would get severely stressed out. During the summer when most of his practice members were on vacation, he'd get mad that they would miss their appointments. His stress level was so high that he literally drove away close to 20 employees in three years. He was so busy trying to control everything that he was missing a terrific opportunity: to take a much-needed break.

One day we were on the phone, and I asked him to stand up. Once he got up, I asked him to squat down as low as he could go, and then jump up as high as he possibly could. I told him not to stop until he reached the clouds. He chuckled and didn't even try to jump. When I asked him why he was laughing, he told me that my request was ridiculous. I said, "I know it is ridiculous, but go ahead and do it anyway. Jump up and touch the clouds."

He jumped and obviously within one second, his feet were back on the ground. When I asked him why he came back to the ground, he laughed again and said, "gravity."

"Are you angry at gravity?" I asked him. He said, "Of course not. I can't control the forces of gravity."

Trying to control all of the things that are out of your control is like trying to control gravity. Accepting the things that are out of your control and facing the reality of them will open the door to exciting opportunities. This simple conversation was life changing to him because now, instead of getting angry when his entire town is on vacation, he vacations during that time himself. He has turned it into great Play Time. He gets the rest, pleasure and enjoyment of wonderful vacations without losing any real productivity, and he is much more energized and focused when he returns to work. The quality of the care he provides has improved dramatically because he is well rested and able to give his all to his patients. What used to be a very difficult and challenging time for him has become a great opportunity, just because he changed his perspective. He made a lobule jump and is taking the new action steps to match.

Part of our internal struggle is that we grow up learning to think about things a certain way. We cling to a lot of our early beliefs even when it is no longer in our best interest to do so. I have a client, a highly successful businessperson with a family of her own, who is now caring for her ailing mother. Unfortunately, her mother is overly critical of her. There is a part of this woman that still values her mother's opinion more than her own. I said to her, "You are 50 years old. At some point, you are going to have to decide that your mother's opinion is just her opinion and you are entitled to one too.

You have to decide if your opinion is the same as your mother's or father's, or if it going to be different. My opinion is that you're a really good person, a really talented person, and a really successful person."

Which opinion do you choose to believe? Which one do you want to nurture for the rest of your life? The one that says you can have fun and enjoy an active, healthy, prosperous life for 100 years and beyond or the one that says you are already old, getting older by the second, and you will end up in a nursing home? Why do we make the negative more important than the positive and exciting? What an unnecessary energy drain that stifles our environment and keeps us from seeing all the opportunities that are right under our noses. Instead, we should place our energy and focus on the compelling vision we wish to create as we customize our ideal 100 Year Lifestyle.

THE ISSUE ABOUT OUR ISSUES

We all have issues. I've learned this from taking care of thousands of patients from all walks of life. I've taken care of celebrities, royalty, professional athletes, and multimillionaires as well as many everyday people. I've taken care of healthy people who were committed to Lifestyle Care and I've also taken care of people who were really sick and suffering. It is amazing how different people respond to their issues, and we all have them—all of us.

The question you have to ask yourself as you change your internal environment is: Do you want to make your issues your life? Or do you want to make your life your life? The people who are having the most fun—and are also the most successful at reaching their goals and achieving balance—are the ones who manage their issues while they live their ideal life. They make their life more important than their issues. They are able to keep things in a perspective that makes inner peace, fulfillment, and happiness more important than their challenges.

Developing a compelling vision for your 100 Year Lifestyle is crucial to your long-term success, health, and happiness and shifts your energy off your issues. Not doing this has been one of the biggest challenges for many of our current seniors and centenarians. Because they didn't know they were going to live as long as they have, many of them have developed destructive, survival, or complacency thought patterns that are causing them to deteriorate way before they should.

Changing your view of longevity from a 60-year or 70-year lifestyle to The 100 Year Lifestyle changes the way you view your life. Develop a vision for your extended life and then change your external environment to match.

When my father got sick with Alzheimer's, everyone in my family was in denial about his condition. My mother, on the other hand, because she lived with him every day, knew that his condition was progressing rapidly. Her ability to accept her situation enabled her to make the best choices to deal with her issues, and live her life. She handled her issues and my dad's issues with class and a proactive approach, while she also lived her life.

While we all watched him deteriorate, we also watched her take the lead on the action steps necessary that, in the long run, were the best for him and the best for her—even though those decisions were difficult ones. What was amazing to me was that during this process, she continued to try and live her best life and make choices that were through progress, not perfection, taking her down the best road for all of us who were involved.

My father has now passed and my mother holds a position that enables her to use her skills as an adult educator. She is making a difference for others and helping people reach their full potential, which is her primary purpose in life. She transitioned from a high-stress intense commute to now working closer to home. She remained loyal and loving to him for nearly 50 years of marriage and through his illness, while using her talents to make a difference as an educator— creating programs for seniors that improve their quality of life.

> **Centenarian Secret**
> To be able to accept your current situation while you also remain committed to creating your compelling future, one choice at a time, is a tremendous skill to develop.

At some of our seminars, we do a hiking session that is all about personal breakthroughs. At one event in particular, I remember going for a walk with a group of seminar attendees at Stone Mountain Park just outside of Atlanta. We climbed up Stone Mountain and when we reached the top, we could see for miles. The landscape was illuminated at certain angles by thousands of homes. Their rooftops penetrated the sky at all different heights. I realized that day that inside every one of those buildings was a reality, a vision, a way of viewing the world that differed in big or small ways from my own as well as from each other. Each reality was defined not only by a unique set of values, experiences, and ambitions, but also by a unique approach to life.

It became clear to me that day, that it is generally more important what happens inside the four walls of each house than outside. What the owner of each house sees from the inside is the only thing he or she can manifest on the outside.

Think about what happens at seven in the morning when the multimillionaire and the construction worker wake up and go to work each day. Both are honorable people with different experiences and views of the world. They breathe the same air, drink the same water and live in the same state. Because they have different visions for their life, they manifest different results in their life.

How about two people in different homes that both make $50,000 a year, and one is in debt up to his eyeballs and one is investing in himself every month. Depending on the vision you see for your life, you will manifest what your mind can see. The internal environment you choose to see will take you as far as you are willing to go. Why not choose to see your ideal 100 Year Lifestyle?

TAP INTO YOUR CREATIVITY

You have to be able to see your life as active, healthy, prosperous, and fun for 100 years in order to create a vision that is compelling. What would be a really exciting and fun life to live for the next 50 years? Begin to talk about it with your life partner, your friends, and your colleagues. Start to voice your vision and bring it into your consciousness. Putting words to it and continuing a dialogue will help you gain the clarity you need to attract the resources, people, and things you need to transition yourself from your current environment to your new one.

We've all heard of the expression "think outside the box." This is lobule jumping. This is an important part of changing your internal and external environment. Drive around different neighborhoods and office parks and look at the various signs, houses, cars, and everything related to environments that are different from yours, but ones you would like to experience. Begin to ask yourself, how do these people think that is different from the way I think?

Start asking questions that open your mind to being able to create a new experience for yourself. Open up to these new possibilities and begin to envision how you can change your environment and make it ideal.

Don't just ask yourself, however; get to know people who can be mentors for you at your stage of life. One thing I have learned about people who are winning in life is that they are usually very willing to help out others who are seriously committed to changing their lives. It's all about intent and the reasons behind your motivation. Widen your scope—think outside of yourself and find a greater purpose—and like the magnets of Life Changing Principle Number 1, you will begin to attract more good things with ease. Being self-righteous and self-centered will repel new and exciting opportunities that are right under your nose. Think about a camera lens. A wide-angle lens expands your field of vision. Be willing to change your internal environment and look through a bigger lens.

LIVE LONG AND STRONG EXERCISE
Think like a champion. List five key attitudes that you can cultivate immediately to attract your ideal 100 Year Lifestyle:
1._____
2._____
3._____
4._____
5._____

What are five activities that you can think of doing right now to cultivate those attitudes? Universal examples might be finding a mentor, forming a mastermind group with high-achieving people who are embracing these 100 Year Lifestyle concepts, joining a neighborhood association and getting involved in activities that improve your community, attending a seminar, participating in a community development project through work, or joining a civic organization.
1._____
2._____
3._____

List at least ten goals that would be exciting to achieve over the next decade.

1. _____
2. _____
3. _____
4. _____
5. _____
6. _____
7. _____
8. _____
9. _____
10. _____

List at least ten things you would absolutely love to do before you turn 100. If you want to list 100 things, go for it. I encourage you to do this. Start a journal and call it 100 Year goals and then fill it up.

1. _____
2. _____
3. _____
4. _____
5. _____
6. _____
7. _____

CHAPTER 13

BALANCING YOUR INTERNAL AND EXTERNAL ENVIRONMENTS

In the first edition of The 100 Year Lifestyle, this chapter was the hardest one for me to write. When I initially went through the manuscript, I completed every chapter and was ecstatic about them. When I got to this chapter, I wrote a fragmented outline and could not really get the flow going. No matter how hard I tried, I got stuck. I flew through the rest of the book and created what I believed was very compelling, life-changing content. But then I had to go back to this one.

It drove me crazy that I could not get this chapter done, knowing how important environment is to The 100 Year Lifestyle.

Finally I realized what the problem was. My external environment was stagnant. It was stifling me. It was cluttered. It wasn't fresh. It had an accumulation of stuff that was no longer significant to me and was just taking up space. There were old clothes stuffed in our closets that were out of style and didn't fit right anymore. There were old books, lots of them, filling up shelves, desktops, and floors. There were numerous repairs that needed to be made to the house, along with several unfinished projects. We had been talking about moving for the last few years and left our environment in limbo, along with this chapter. I had to fix my own external environment first before I could tackle this text.

I declared a family workday and Lisa, the kids, and I went on a cleansing binge. We freed up the space—throwing out 100 big bags of garbage, giving away 20 bags of clothes, and 11 boxes of books to charity.

After that, this chapter came together for me instantly on the day that I declared our family workday and committed to cleansing our environment. Change really is much easier than thinking about change.

Is your environment stifling to you? Or is it the one that you can enjoy for the balance of your years? Do you have a dozen incomplete projects lying around? How are they impacting your energy? Are you feeling stuck?

Take action immediately by changing your external environment. Start with where you are and begin to cleanse. Cleaning up your environment opens up the space for new, exciting ideas and opportunities that will free your creative spirit and bring freshness into your life.

For my family, this cleansing opened up a lot of exciting opportunities for all of us. Our vision for our life and environment has been creatively inspired. We are more excited about entertaining again and sharing our beautiful home with friends and family. We are more relaxed during our Play Time when we are at home. Our chronic stress has gone down, which has freed up energy for other opportunities. We have opened up more vision-oriented discussions within our family and it has been very rewarding for all of us. Making the changes sure is easier than thinking about making them.

Living The 100 Year Lifestyle: The Immersion Experience

The Immersion Experience will really help you shift your life, family, practice, business to new levels of enjoyment, fulfillment and success. Why? Because you will stop dabbling, and immerse yourself.

Fully immersing yourself into your 100 Year Lifestyle will increase your attractor factor exponentially.

LIVE LONG AND STRONG EXERCISE

Define your ideal home environment: _____

_____

What is currently missing from this environment that you would like to change or add? _____

_____

Define your ideal work environment _____

_____

What is currently missing from this environment that you would like to change or add? _____

_____

What changes do you need to make to create the ideal environment you can enjoy for 100 years? _____

_____

What unfinished projects do you need to complete or let go of? _____

_____

TRANSITION STRATEGIES TO CHANGE YOUR ENVIRONMENT

One way of reducing stress caused by your environment is to get in the habit of completing activities that you begin. I have a good friend who has ten major projects going on at once in his home and it is really causing a lot of stress to his family. Loose ends can make you lose your mind.

Consider stimulating your environment with music and spending less time in front of the television. With digital video recorders, internet TV and YouTube, it is so easy and inexpensive these days to filter through the television muck and fill your life with the few shows that are important to you. Of course, you can also watch them at a time that is convenient for you, rather than rushing to catch your favorite show before it starts. In today's day and age, television begins when you want it to and you can turn it off whenever you want also.

Further, make sure your environment is in line with your personality. When Lisa and I moved into our first home, we invested a lot of money to decorate it. We were young and excited, and we decided on a style that was exactly like our parents' style. While the décor was first-class and nice, we realized a few months later that while it was beautiful, it wasn't our style. As you gain maturity—which is the beauty of being able to begin life again with 40, 50, or 60 years' experience—you really begin to connect with your own style. From the clothes you wear to the colors in your home, you can totally change the look and feel of your life by connecting with your Innate Intelligence, cultivating a willingness to think outside your box and experimenting with different styles.

Also, reconsider time that you "don't have any control over." For instance, not too long ago, one of my patients took a new job that required her to spend a total of two hours in her vehicle commuting to and from work. While the job alleviated some of her financial stress, it added to her emotional and mental stress. In fact, the aggravation and anxiety that accompanied sitting in traffic became so acute that it interfered with her ability to work once she finally got into the office.

I helped her see this new circumstance as an opportunity. I pointed out to her that an hour each way translated into ten hours a week, or 520 hours a year of time that she now had to develop her knowledge and skills in any area that she was passionate about. She could use the time to meditate, listen to self-help or motivational recordings, learn a language, enjoy an audio book, or tutor herself in business or other area of interest. Soon, she began to see this time as a resource and as an opportunity for growth. She no longer let her commute time cause her stress.

She has since quit her job and started a home-based business using her core talents and she combines them with many of the concepts she learned while commuting. What an opportunity her commute turned out to be. She stimulated her internal environment to make changes in her external environment, which created a cycle of change that improved her life dramatically. You are doing the exact same thing by reading this book. You are stimulating your internal environment, which will cause you to take action and start living your ideal 100 Year Lifestyle.

EXPERIENCES THAT YOU GIVE YOURSELF

Try changing your external environment from the drug store to the health food store. You'd be amazed at how many millions of people who used to depend on drugs for everyday living now just choose to eat healthier, take supplements, get chiropractic Lifestyle Care, and exercise regularly to ensure they are as healthy as possible.

Change your environment from a fast-food restaurant to a healthy alternative. Drive to the gym instead of the mall. Rearrange your furniture. Change things up and begin to view the world a little differently to stimulate your creativity.

Destructive patterns in your environment reinforce your current life. For example, driving to the liquor store on your way home each night will ensure that you drink. Going out for ice cream every night will ensure that you continue to pack on the pounds. Replace these destructive energy patterns with new human potential patterns and support them with healthy, 100 Year Lifestyle environment choices.

This is why your shopping patterns are important. Remember when you are food shopping that what you buy is even more important than what you eat, because you will eat what you buy. Where you shop is also important because if you shop in a food store that sells organic groceries, you will bring healthier choices into your home. Since the first edition of The 100 Year Lifestyle was published, the numbers of healthy, organic and green options have grown significantly, giving you more choices and creating a more competitive market.

A common mistake we make is to try to prove to ourselves that we are past our old habits by pushing ourselves back into negative patterns and trying to resist them. As an example, alcoholics who go back into the bars to prove they won't drink are more likely to go back to their addiction. If you go back to the same patterns, before you know it, you'll be back to the same routine, suffering from the same challenges as before. You'll know that you're really "past" something when you have shut the door on it forever and don't feel the urge to look back. This is a sign of real change.

LIVE LONG AND STRONG EXERCISE
Begin to define your ideal environment:
Describe your ideal home environment _____

_____

Describe your ideal work environment _____

_____

Describe your ideal vacation environment _____

_____

Create an external environment that resonates with your internal environment and supports your human potential pattern. Take all of your old memorabilia in your home that is no longer relevant or supportive of the next phase of your life and box it up. If it is relevant but a part of your history, move it to a designated place in your home where you keep all of your past. Designate this area as your personal museum, and fill the rest of your environment with things that inspire your future or help you make the most enjoyment out of the present. Do the same thing at work by filling your environment with elements that enhance a positive and productive attitude. When you enjoy your space at home, at work, in your car, and in your daily activities, you will feed the lifestyle you deserve and desire.

BE CONGRUENT INSIDE AND OUT

The key is to create an external environment that is congruent with your internal one. This congruency will give you peace of mind, keep you centered, and establish an environment and lifestyle that is uniquely important to you. When your internal and external environment are not congruent, the consequences can be destructive.

I noticed an example of incongruence one day when I saw a beautiful Mercedes convertible stopped at a traffic light with the music blasting. At first glance I noticed the car and said to myself, "Wow, that's a beautiful car." Then I thought to myself, "That person must be very successful." Finally, I looked through the window and saw a 300-pound man crammed into the driver seat with the steering wheel pressing a two-inch indent in his stomach. I wondered how he got in there. I wondered how he gets out. And how on earth does he drive with the steering wheel wedged against his bulging abdomen? This unfortunate soul is headed for a serious crisis and I'm not sure which will come first, the car accident or the heart attack. I wonder how long he will be able to enjoy that beautiful automobile.

Additional areas of incongruence can be living above your means, tolerating abusive relationships, eating healthy or starving yourself all day and binging at night, and compromising your voice by not speaking up when you know you have something valuable to say.

Congruency with your internal environment and your external one will help you create your ideal 100 Year Lifestyle and give you the inner peace to enjoy the journey every step of the way.

LIVE LONG AND STRONG EXERCISE
Identify areas of incongruence between your internal environment and your external environment: _____

_____

How are they affecting you? _____
The immediate thoughts and actions you can take to create congruency are: _____

As you do the Live Long and Strong exercises throughout this book you will probably begin to notice a pattern of things to do that repeat themselves over and over again. This is exciting because you will realize that the closer you get to your core, the simpler it is to transition your environment and make the changes that you know you need to make. Start having more fun than ever by committing to the internal and external environments that feed your mind, body, and spirit. You already know what to do. Trust your Innate Intelligence. Now that you feel better, have more energy, and have begun to change your environment, let's begin to attract the right people into our lives and build on our experiences so that we maximize our enjoyment in the next phase of our extended lives.

CARING FOR OUR GLOBAL ENVIRONMENT

What's the point in living to 100 if there is not going to be a planet to live on? Let's spend a few minutes talking about this environment that we all share. As the world's population continues to grow, the impact of this growth is likely to catch up to us. I think again of my 300-pound friend driving the beautiful Mercedes who was busting out of his space. As the world's population grows, it is more important than ever that we live in sync with our environment and not put short-term gains ahead of our collective long-term health.

Let's be quality-of-life motivated versus crisis motivated when it comes to our natural resources. We know we all want to breathe clean air and drink clean water. We all want to enjoy the oceans, mountains, lakes, and streams. Every choice we make affects our environment—from the way we dispose of our waste products to the items we buy in the store. Green buildings are "in" because responsible builders are realizing that people want to be in an environment that is healthy. And what is healthy for us is also healthy for our environment.

"Green" is now mainstream and thank goodness. Green construction by definition is quality construction—no corners are cut, and waste is kept to a minimum. Learn about builders in your area that specialize in green building and learn about their certification and knowledge.

"Green" homes rival "smart" homes in terms of awe-inspiring features and amenities like geothermal heating and windows with photo-chromatic glazing, which grow darker to block out heat in the summer, but stay clear in winter. "You see the shift toward green through the number of green products now making their way into the marketplace," says Steven Kleber, the head of a marketing firm in Atlanta specializing in products for the home. "We've seen a change not only in terms of the sheer volume of products, but also in terms of their variation and the number of companies entering the market. Many of our best-known companies will eventually tap this market."

Recently I went back to visit my alma mater, Life University, and was blown away at their Socrates Café, the benchmark in Green dining in a university setting. The key thing to remember is that you don't have to uproot your life to be green. There are a million and one little things you can start doing today to protect the environment. They include recycling, turning off lights, and installing a dehumidifier on your central AC system to pull moisture out of the air in the summer—allowing you to cool more efficiently. If you are building a home, look into construction materials and most importantly, builders that work in sync with the environment. Like the titration experiment we discussed in Life Changing Principle Number 2, every drop counts!

THE 100 YEAR LIFESTYLE
ACTION PLAN FOR LASTING CHANGE

1. Have gratitude and appreciate your current environment. Look for the good right where you are, and make the most of your current environment. If you are not willing to take the time to begin constructing your compelling future in your current environment, you will probably re-create the past in your new one if you move.

2. Begin to develop your vision for your ideal 100 Year Lifestyle environment. Verbalize your dreams with people who are close to you, who you trust to support you in creating it. Keep a journal of the things that are important to you for your internal and external environment. Continue to define and redefine, with more and more clarity, your ideal 100 Year Lifestyle.

3. Begin to train yourself to think outside the box and magnetically attract what you want. Catch yourself when your thoughts move into destructive patterns and immediately shift yourself back to your ideal mindset.

4. Let go of trying to control the things that are out of your control and focus on the things that you truly can change. Through this acceptance and letting go process you will begin to formulate a transition strategy that will help you change your environment.

5. Describe your ideal home and work environments. Identify any changes that you can immediately make to improve your environment and make it more enjoyable.

6. Start having more fun and enjoying the journey now. Look for the good in every situation. Choose to make your life more fun. Appreciate your progress at this point in your life and the lessons you have learned along the way. They have set the stage for you to maximize the rest of your 100 years.

7. Be good to the planet. Become environmentally conscious and encourage your family and friends to do the same. We are all in this together.

LIVE LONG AND STRONG EXERCISE
List three things you can start doing today to live more in sync with your environment:
1._____
2._____
3._____

PART 6

Building a Rock Solid Support System You Can Enjoy For 100 Years

Nobody wants to get to 100 years old alone.

CHAPTER 14

CONNECTING WITH MULTIPLE GENERATIONS AND CIRCLES OF PEOPLE

By this stage of the game, you know what's best for your health and your environment. These are key components of enjoying a quality 100 years because nobody wants to age suffering the consequences of pain, sickness, and disease, while also living in an unpleasant environment that is out of their control or incongruent with their Innate Intelligence. In my interviews with people all over the world, another key concern that people have about aging is loneliness.

NOBODY WANTS TO GET TO 100 YEARS OLD ALONE

This chapter is all about creating a rock solid support system that you can enjoy for 100 years. I call this the Surround Sound System of Support. This type of support system enhances the quality of our lives and our experiences—just like our home entertainment centers enhance our enjoyment of music and movies. This is extremely important for you today–and even more important for you as you age. Study after study has shown that strong social relationships are essential for a healthy mind and body, while also enhancing our life experience. They reduce some of the bad effects of stress, and help speed recovery from psychological and physical illness. They also support our desire for longevity. After all, nobody wants to make it to next year alone, not to mention to age 100. Supportive relationships sustain us and help us to maximize our enjoyment in life.

Here are 9 areas or circles where you can immediately begin to look for and build your 100 Year Lifestyle relationships:

1. Religious, spiritual
2. Family
3. Friends
4. Sports
5. Hobbies
6. Politics
7. Education
8. Travel
9. Causes

The *Journal of the American Medical Association* recently reported on a study in which several hundred volunteers were exposed to a cold virus. The study showed that the volunteers with the most socially diverse networks were the most disease resistant—only 35 percent of the volunteers with six or more close relationships caught the cold. But 65 percent of the volunteers with three or fewer close relationships caught it. You may have also read the recent study showing the potent, positive effect that support groups have on breast cancer patients, improving their healing ability. It is exciting news to know that good support is not only more fun, but it also makes a difference. It's exciting to know that so many factors that affect our quality of life are under our control.

A Surround Sound Support System is really pretty easy to create. However, it's going to require an investment of time.

Let's begin with the relationship you have with yourself. As I'm sure you've heard before, this is one of the most important relationships you'll ever have outside of your relationship with your Maker. The way you treat yourself is reflected in all of your key relationships. You magnetically attract people and circumstances into your life based on the energy and effort you put into nurturing them. If you ever wake up one day and realize that you've ended up in the wrong relationship, or the right relationship gone wrong, and it is time to make a change, the place to start is with you.

We've all heard the expression "You teach people how to treat you." They watch how you treat yourself and learn from you how you like to be treated. If you are surrounded by people who are abusive to you, ask yourself, "Am I one of them?" One of the things you may notice is that if you have implemented the strategies on energy we have discussed, stopped destructive habits that were killing you, adopted the Health Care Hierarchy, and implemented a self-care and health care regimen, wrongs that others have committed against you will begin to stand out like a sore thumb. They will become more noticeable and intolerable to you, just like the person who finally quits smoking detests the smell of cigarette smoke.

Centenarian Secret

Understand that healthy relationships are created and adaptive. Connect with the people in your world in a way that is authentic. Expect that some of your relationships will change over time. Let it happen. Continue to add people to your life who support the healthiest side of you. Discern who has your best interests at heart and make yourself one of those people.

START BY SUPPORTING YOURSELF

Many people don't realize we have the power to attract into our lives exactly what we need. You attract what you need by nurturing yourself and staying true to your Innate—by being authentic. Don't look for someone else to make things better for you. Take action while you also express your true nature.

One of our 100 Year Lifestyle Affiliate chiropractors runs her own practice, is a single mom, and the breadwinner for her family. While she has established a great practice that is providing great quality care for the people in her community, she was always trying to figure out how to handle everything and bring her life back into balance. She kept looking outside herself for support, but she was never able to find exactly what she needed. She kept hoping that a knight in shining armor would show up and save her. She felt that she needed outside support to get things under control and even said several times, "I don't know how much longer I can handle all of this."

One day, in a phone conversation, I told her, "You're not going to get the support you need until you are willing to support yourself." I then asked her to consider this: "If you were the only resource where support existed, what would you do differently today? How would you give yourself the support you need?"

She said, "I'd start my days differently by taking some time for myself early in the morning before the kids get up. When I take my son to baseball practice, I'd exercise instead of simply sitting there—waiting for practice to be over." She also said she would make a staff change because one of her employees was not working up to par, which was draining. This employee was actually creating more work and stress for her.

She said she would also create relationships that would support her in taking care of the kids' activities—including carpools and tutors. She said she would take a vacation and go to a spa at least twice a year to really pamper herself. And she also said that she would spend more time thinking through the upcoming week so that her days would be more focused go more smoothly. At that time, she was kind of randomly attacking her days—with the hopes of surviving another one.

I was amazed by how easy it was for her to come up with so many ideas. She knew what she needed to do. But she was still frantically looking for answers outside of herself. I'm not sure why this happens, but you see this so often. Maybe this is because we live in a society that promises quick fixes for almost everything. So our first reaction in a time of crisis is to grasp for quick-fix solutions, which invariably will make things seem better temporarily while the underlying challenges persist. Instead of attracting the support you need, you end up repelling it. Sometimes the rock solid support arrives in a form that you weren't expecting and you end up rejecting it.

When you are crisis oriented only and creating lots of stress, your mind can become easily distracted from all the good. As a result, you miss opportunities and solutions that are right in front of you. This is why it is so important to nurture yourself—especially during times of transition. When you focus on attracting solutions instead of scrambling to grasp for them, you are receptive to the good stuff that will invariably come your way naturally. Building on that is how you will ultimately transition to a better place and attract the support you desire.

LIVE LONG AND STRONG

If you were the only person in your life where support existed, what would you change immediately to ensure that you get the support you need:

1. _____
2. _____
3. _____
4. _____
5. _____

SUPPORT YOURSELF THROUGH YOUR CHOICES

Once you know how to support yourself—which for many of us takes the first 30, 40, or 50 years of our lives—it becomes easier to ask for the right type of support from others. You may be the kind of person who needs quiet time. Ask for it. You may need to exercise in a way that's different from your partner. Go for it. Take it. Do the things that you need to do for yourself and you'll discover that you have so much more to give to your relationships.

SUPPORT YOURSELF: ESTABLISH A PERSONAL RENEWAL RECIPE

Have you ever returned home from a vacation and felt completely refreshed? Have you ever said to someone you love, "I feel like a new person"? Well, what were you doing when that happened? What made you feel that way? *What if you set up your life with this renewal in mind?*

Wouldn't it be great if your work gave you a sense of renewal, fed your passion, and stimulated your mind as well as your pocketbook? Wouldn't it be exciting if the rest of your daily routines did the same? Making personal renewal a part of your lifestyle is what will surely keep your mind, body, and spirit young, regardless of your age.

SUPPORT AND RENEW YOUR BODY THROUGH MOVEMENT

A great first action when you wake up in the morning is to move every joint in your body. Stand up straight with your feet together and breathe in—as deep as you can. Hold it in for five seconds. Feel the air enter spaces in your lungs you don't normally utilize. As the air enters, raise your arms above your head. After five seconds, blow the air out hard while you lower your arms—again to the count of five.

Repeat this exercise five times with your eyes closed and then begin to move every part of your body—one at a time, beginning with the top of your head. Roll your eyes in a clockwise direction and then reverse. Do the same with your neck, slowly rolling it in a full range of motion and then reversing it. Do each direction three to five times. Scrunch up all your facial muscles by making a lot of funny faces and then release them.

This may seem silly, but most of us aren't utilizing our bodies to anywhere near their capabilities. This creates a state of imbalance and disharmony inside us. We are made to move through much greater ranges of motion than our twenty-first-century lives call for. When you start the day stretching this way, you will wake up your entire body and feel energized instantly.

Continue stretching your way throughout your body. Include your shoulders, elbows, wrists, fingers, chest, waist, upper and lower spine, hips, knees, feet, and toes. If you like the feeling you get from this type of full-body movement, yoga would be a fantastic exercise for you.

Every cell of your body will begin to wake up, and you'll like it. The cracks that you hear will remind you that you are not a kid. Keep in mind that your healthful movements are slowing down the aging process as you work out all the kinks. You might inform your chiropractor, massage therapist, or personal trainer about the places you feel the most kinked up so they can help you work through it and help you rebuild your body in the healthiest and best way.

Go through these motions two to three times a day and they will keep your body awake and regenerated. It only takes five minutes and the awakening will help you feel alive.

I remember when I attended a car control clinic with my son Jacob when he was fifteen, after he received his learner's permit. One key point made by the instructor is that most driving is done without turning the wheel through its full range of motion. The average turn only takes the wheel through a half to one full revolution. This becomes a habit for most of us and especially for teenagers. Young drivers are actually often afraid to really turn the wheel all the way, which can sometimes cause them to experience unnecessary accidents.

When I heard this, I thought automatically of the way many of us treat our bodies. Our lives have grown so sedentary. We forget the multitude of tasks that our bodies are capable of doing. Every day we hear stories of 85, 90 and even 100 year old people who are running races, climbing mountains and performing extraordinary tasks. A very important aspect of The 100 Year Lifestyle is to have confidence in your body so it can support you with any activity you choose. Making personal renewal a part of your lifestyle will give you the body confidence you need throughout every phase of your life.

While you may not be able to feel like you are 18 again, you'll be amazed at how youthful, active, and healthy you'll feel by making renewal a part of your daily life. If you ask anyone who feels old what makes them feel that way, they will often tell you that they can no longer do the things that they want to do. Their capabilities are less than they would like. You can get much of this youthful physical feeling back with full-body movement.

You also renew your body and mind through rest. Getting enough sleep, and getting quality sleep, is important. Have the right bed and pillow to support your spine and nervous system is vital to your wellbeing. If you share your bed with a life partner and you have different shapes, both of you should be able to customize your side of the mattress. You both deserve the right support for you. Also, if you sit for long periods of time at work, get an ergonomic chair to support your back.

Take the self-care and health care strategies that work best for you and put them into your daily routine, and you will customized your Personal Renewal Recipe.

MAGNETICALLY ATTRACTING AN ABUNDANCE OF SUPPORT

The next level of support comes from family and close friends. We often tend to take these relationships for granted. Just like the relationships with ourselves, we overlook their importance. However, you'll find that the quality of your life will skyrocket when you invest in the relationships that are closest to home.

Today, ask your partner, "What are the changes you want to make in your life? How can I support you?" Switch. Take turns. Really listen to your partner and then follow through to make those changes a part of your lifestyle. As a couple ask, "What are the changes we know we need to make? What action step can we undertake today to make those changes part of our new 100 Year Lifestyle?" Give each other the opportunity to voice what is important and then support each other in making the changes you know you that you need to make.

Your primary relationship has a major impact on your health. Studies have documented the health and economic benefits of a happy marriage and they have also chronicled the cost of an unhappy marriage, divorce, and death. Studies have determined that divorce and widowhood create stress, which has been linked to chronic health problems. Couples or singles who live with aging parents or grandkids often showed negative consequences, in terms of their physical, cognitive, or emotional health, especially if their primary relationship is not strong. Keeping your primary relationship strong is essential to the quality of life you want and deserve.

The next level of Surround Sound Support is to connect with people who have interests that are similar to yours. Look for them while pursuing some of your favorite activities—like attending worship services, traveling, mentoring, spending time with friends, and working. Lean on them for support and offer them support as well.

A SURROUND SOUND SUPPORT SYSTEM FOR YOUR MIND, BODY, AND SPIRIT

A Surround Sound System of Support covers all of your bases. You should have people in your life who support you in pursuing the quality of life that you desire, in reaching your full potential, and in helping you through crises.

When you look at your current support system, you may find that you have support only for times of crisis. When this happens, you might find yourself on an emotional roller coaster. This should not be the primary way that you connect with people. Think of it this way: If your financial advisor specializes in debt relief, you will struggle to build wealth because you won't have the proper support in place. If you have a doctor who only treats disease, you won't have all the information you need to achieve optimum health over your extended life.

Surrounding yourself with the right type of support is very freeing for your soul, because you know you'll be able to make the best of every situation. Discuss your long-term vision and also be a good listener. Healthy relationships are a two way street.

MULTIPLE CIRCLES AND GENERATIONS OF RELATIONSHIPS

One of the greatest fears and challenges of aging is loneliness and being alone. When we are younger and surrounded by children, their youthful energy can be contagious and make us feel young. There are a lot of birthdays to attend, anniversaries to celebrate, births, confirmations, bar mitzvahs, and many other opportunities to celebrate. Our calendars are filled with celebrations of the joys of being alive, with an occasional funeral thrown into the mix. This type of balance makes it easier to stay positive and motivated on a daily basis. These celebrations make life fun.

For many in our current generation of seniors and centenarians, they unfortunately experience more funerals than parties. When speaking to Papa Hy about this before he died, he told me about how sad he was when one of his pinochle friends had recently passed. They used to sit around and play cards together for hours on a regular basis. He missed their playful interactions and friendship.

The imbalance between celebrations and sadness can lead to depression and hopelessness as you age. Loss is going to be a reality of our extended life spans. The longer you live, the more loss you will experience. Unbalanced loss without celebrations to offset them can create numerous challenges, including feelings of loneliness or depression. If you only have one circle of friends, or one friend, you will put yourself in a position to be extremely depressed in the event of a significant loss. The more circles you have, and the more places in which you are meaningfully connected, the easier it is going to be for you to enjoy your longevity. You will be more able to cope with loss and stay passionately engaged in life.

I remember when we hosted a huge weekend celebration in honor of my son Cory's thirteenth birthday. Papa Hy flew up from Florida to be with us, and when he got there, he looked every second of his 99 years. By the time he left, he looked at least 15 years younger. Being around a multiple generations of people, while also participating in this celebration, really brought back his youthful energy.

Certainly, grief is a part of the process of loss but when your life is multidimensional, it is easier to move forward. Building relationships with three, four, even five generations of people balances you and stimulates your youthfulness. When you maintain relationships across generations, you stay in touch with the radically changing world in which we live. This keeps your senses young and sharp. It keeps you active and alive.

Centenarian Secret
Learn from the experience and wisdom of the mature and share the passion and zest for life of the young.

Further, don't overlook the value of purpose. Seniors who are retired and not involved in a profession, religious organization, or a volunteer group are at a higher risk of health problems, including depression. Staying involved in things that are important to you will give you a reason to get up every morning. Having several reasons to get up is even more important and much healthier than having a one-dimensional life without a lot of support. The more you give to multiple generations and multiple circles of people, the more support that will come back to you when you need it at times of loss.

RESTRUCTURED FAMILIES

Treasure the relationships closest to you—even if they come in a form that you weren't expecting. Restructured families are becoming the norm. They tend to take shape with a lot of emotional baggage. You may have experienced this in your own life—or in the life of one of your children. Many people have a tendency to pull back from these types of relationships and resist the change intensely.

What would happen instead if you refrained from judging too much in these situations and reached out to your new family? While I would not want you to compromise your loyalties, I would encourage you to develop bonds with children brought in by a new marriage, for example. It is going to become important for us to accept our extended families and develop relationships with their extended families. *Harmony within these relationships is essential and can eliminate a lot of unnecessary stress.*

These families are not going away. They are going to be a part of our lives for the rest of our lives. Accepting this and treating each other with mutual respect, love, support, and admiration is going to be important to ensure the quality of life we desire for 80, 90, 100 years and beyond. To resist this is a complete energy drain, like resisting gravity, as we saw earlier. Why create this extra stress in what can already be a stressful situation? Why waste the energy trying to control others or being self-righteous about our anger and disconnectedness?

Relationships with stepchildren and step-grandchildren can enhance the quality of your life and can assist you in developing a support system for your present and future. What you put out comes back to you. You can't expect to receive down the road if you don't give the support now. Understand that we can choose the amount of time we spend with these people and the level of involvement they have in our lives. But to deny their existence and push those relationships away just perpetuates separation and pain.

Centenarian Secret
Our generation will be the first in a history to have five generations in a family as the norm. We will get to know our family tree with more depth beginning with the newborn baby, 25-year-old parents, 50-year-old grandparents, 75-year-old great-grandparents, and 100 year-old great-great-grandparents.

Multiple generations are going to have to learn to get along, work together, and support each other for the good of society as a whole. How can we do this? How do we balance our old-world values with the technological advances in this high-paced, rapidly changing world? To do so requires an understanding and appreciation of generations outside our own.

One evening when we had our parents over for dinner, we were talking around the table about this very issue. I ended up, accidentally, hurting my father's feelings when I said that he was old-fashioned. But I meant it as a compliment. I have realized that old-fashioned values like prioritizing family, being spiritually grounded, and having a good work ethic, name, and reputation are very important to an individual's success in life, and to the foundation of our culture. What is also important to him, however, is the adventurousness that comes from a youthful mind. Blending these values and accepting the gifts that each generation has to offer can build relationships that keep the older generations younger and energetic while keeping the younger generations wise beyond their years. For the older generations, they connect them to celebrations—from births to birthday parties to confirmations, graduations, and weddings.

Papa Hy—when he was 99—looked forward to special events with his great-grandchildren with so much pleasure. You can connect to these types of events through your family and extended family—as well as through churches and synagogues, professional groups, hobbies, and areas of activism with which you are affiliated. To benefit from these circles of generations you've got to be willing to show up and attend. Be there and participate with authenticity and genuine goodwill.

Multiple circles might include professional, sports, religious, friendship, family, support groups, and others. I have seen people get consumed with one circle and neglect the others, causing an imbalance, boredom, and stress. Your Quality Time Calendar will provide you with the structure to help you achieve this balance in your life.

You may find from time to time that some of your support systems run dry. You veer away from the values shared by certain circles of friends. They no longer seem like viable components of your rock solid support system and you might consider letting them go. Disconnecting is always an option, but so is changing your expectations.

For example, if alcohol is a destructive pattern, you may need to disconnect from the bar scene. If you wish to settle down, you may start to disconnect from the singles' scene. Alternatively, if your family is not a rock solid support system, but you cannot disconnect from them, you may simply choose to reset your expectations with respect to them. If they are unable or unwilling to give you the support you need, stop looking to them for support.

LIFELONG LEARNING AND MULTIPLE CAREERS

During the first 30, 40 to 50 years of your life you will build the skills to really optimize the last 40 or 50 years. If you are 50 years old today, think about what you knew and what you were learning 50 years ago. Think about it. Fifty years ago you were learning how to suckle milk from a bottle or your mother's bosom. Do you think you've learned a few things since then? Was your learning conscious? Did you choose your learning? During kindergarten through eighth grade, you embraced your environment and got to know how to interact with the other children. You also got to know some basic skills.

In high school you learned how to rebel, along with the skills to get you to college. Maybe you decided to learn a trade. Maybe you didn't learn much at all and just partied your brains out. Either way, you collected experiences that on some level have shaped your life today. In college you learned the skills to land a job or targeted a profession to work in so you could make a living. Now here you are with maybe 40, 50, or 60 years left. Do you think there are a few more things you might like to learn and master over these remaining decades? What would you love to learn? You have plenty of time to get excited about mastering new skills, taking adventures, traveling the world, experiencing different cultures, starting a new business.

Dan Sullivan, the founder and CEO of The Strategic Coach, teaches that you set goals in areas of life that are of interest to you, and in the achievement of those goals, you learn about things that are meaningful to your life. Your goals actually become the foundation for your own personal school of life. What an inspiring way to look at lifelong learning. And if you are an entrepreneur who wants to get the most out of life, you should seriously consider his program.

Embrace multiple generations of family, friends, and community. You will stay engaged in life and build Surround Sound Support to sustain you during your longevity.

When you feel the support it becomes easier to embrace the opportunities that the world has to offer, including new knowledge, skills, and adventures.

What do you want to learn over the next 10, 20, or 30 years? Do you want to master finances? Do you want to learn about real estate? Do you want to learn to ski, hike 14,000 foot mountains, or become an expert in organic gardening? Are you ready to see the world? It's your 100 Year Lifestyle and it's your choice. Let's get excited about a life of constant learning.

CHAPTER 15

EMBRACING YOUR PASSIONS THROUGH LIFELONG LEARNING

Studies show that seniors engaged in artistic pursuits are actually improving their health. But don't pursue lifelong learning and creativity simply to produce longevity, make it a part of your lifestyle so that you make your journey enjoyable and passionate every step of the way. There will be seasons when you're constantly feeding your hunger for knowledge, feeding your creative drive, and cultivating your rock solid support system. You will also have seasons when you are growing your business, and raising your family. There may also be seasons when you relax and beach yourself. Maybe you are or have been in hibernation season, like a bear, and are ready to come out of your cave.

The important thing is to never hold yourself back from change and lifelong learning because you think you are "too old." I'll never forget the first time I heard a 30 year old patients say that to me. It was quite startling. You are never too young or old to learn. New seasons and passions may arrive unexpectedly at times. Embrace them. Take the time to think about all the things you would love to experience in your lifetime. You may be overtaken with a desire to do something out of the box. Seizing such moments is what The 100 Year Lifestyle is all about.

Since the first edition of The 100 Year Lifestyle was published, a fun movie called The Bucket List came out and now it seems like everyone is making this list and checking things off as they go. Your Bucket List can be filled with experiences you want to have, trips you want to take, and things that you would like to learn. You will attract multiple circles and generations of people to support you with the individual items on your list, making great new friends along the way.

Life Changing Principle Number 2 is so important, as the choice to stay in the game and not let the challenges get you down is crucial to enjoying your journey and reaching your goals. You never know which is going to be the final drop of knowledge and experience that makes the biggest impact on you or has the most meaning. Embrace them all with passion.

Letting go of past mistakes is very important for growth and progress. Many people become afraid to learn new things because of previous mistakes. Forgive yourself, and others who may have hurt you, and move on. Learn from them and re-engage. An extreme example of this involved one of my clients. He had been audited and ended up owing the IRS $200,000 in back taxes. It was simply paralyzing him. The government wanted its money paid back in the amount of $25,000 a quarter for the next two years. Unfortunately he was not producing the income necessary to meet these demands. The problem was not his business, however; the problem was in his mind. He was unable to see how this was the lesson he needed to become financially independent. At first, he was unwilling to change his ways. At 48 years of age, he had not saved any money and he was smothered by this debt.

Centenarian Secret

Everyone makes mistakes. The longer you live, the more mistakes you will make. Learn from them. Grow from them. Forgive yourself and others who may have hurt you. Move on.

I instructed him to figure the $200,000 into his overhead, accept his fate, and go to work with a greater sense of purpose than ever before. I got him to see the lesson embedded in this experience. I told him to think of it this way: "If this experience teaches you to expand your business by this amount, after two years you'll have paid off the IRS and you will have an extra $25,000 a quarter to invest toward your future. That's $100,000 a year. By the time you are 60 years old you will have accumulated $1,000,000. Say thank you for the forced lesson, and change your life." As of this time, he is well on his way, and you can be too.

ARE YOU READY FOR YOUR NEXT BIG THING?

Are you still hibernating? Or are you ready for Your Next Big Thing? What would get you excited about the next phase of your life? Choosing Your Next Big Thing will bring incredible passion back into your life. Expose yourself to new and exciting people, and bring the little kid inside of you back out again. Are you ready to come out of your cave and commit to your ideal 100 Year Lifestyle? If not now, when? Open your eyes. See the people who are there to support you. Once you commit to Your Next Big Thing, you will be amazed by how much support you will attract.

No matter what your age is today, there is always a new "Next Big Thing" to commit yourself to—what will it be for you today? A business? A charity? Travel? People you would like to meet? Make a list of Your Next Big Things that you would like to accomplish or experience in your extended life. Meditate or pray over your list for a few weeks and see if you can gain clarity over what Your Next Big Thing is going to be. Commit to it and make it happen. Enjoy the journey along the way. The second you commit to it, your passion will surface and you will feel that youthful energy deep in your gut. You will attract the support you need to make it happen.

I remember when Papa Hy was trying to figure out how to work a VCR and how much he struggled with this simple task. For his generation, change occurred very slowly and technological change was not a cultural phenomenon. It is now! Embracing change as a part of your lifestyle eliminates the frustration that resisting change can create. Technology, for example, is here to stay and the one thing that we can be sure of is that there will constantly be new products, services, and ideas that transform the way we live our lives. We are fortunate to grow up in an age of innovation. Over the course of our 100 Year Lifestyle, we can be sure that this trend will continue. Continue to embrace innovation with a willingness to learn.

What would you like to learn over the next 30, 40, or 50 years of your life? Would you like to learn about wine and food? Would you like to learn about different cultures and visit them all? Would it be exciting for you to learn how to build and sell a company? Would you like to learn how to write a book? Maybe you would like to become a master of healthy relationships and learn how to surround yourself with them. There is no time like the present to begin making the changes that you know you need to make and to start setting exciting new goals, Your Next Big Things!

KEEPING YOURSELF FRESH FOR 100 YEARS AND BEYOND

Make the rest of your life one big thing after another and you will keep that freshness and passion flowing. Fresh energy keeps you young. Stress speeds aging. We have all felt the effects of stress on our bodies during challenging times, and we've all seen how stress causes people to look older. I remember seeing before-and-after pictures of President Clinton's term in office and thinking to myself how much older he looked. I remember the same was true for President Jimmy Carter and President George Bush. Studies on the science of "telomeres" have shown that stress does speed the aging process. Let go and keep learning.

Making lifelong learning a part of your personality keeps you fresh and minimizes the effects of stress while also slowing down the aging process. Explore the latest advances in exercise, information and technology. As your goals change, change up your routines to keep them fresh and in line with your vision. Don't get stuck in a rut of boredom. Change things up. Change is good.

YOUR SIXTH SENSE

Keep your senses stimulated. Science says we have five senses. Intuition is the sixth sense. When your five senses are sharp, your sixth sense will be even sharper, and you will rely on this sixth sense your entire lifetime.

One of my favorite sayings that I learned in Chiropractic college was, "trust your Innate". The book, *Gut Feelings: The Intelligence of the Unconscious* by Gerd Gigerenzer, backs up this mantra. Researchers found that athletes and business people who trusted their gut feeling performed better and got better results. Your sixth sense, your Innate Intelligence, your gut will take care of you.

Centenarian Secret
Keep your senses stimulated by spending time in nature. Notice every small detail, from the sounds of the wind and water to the colors on the leaves and flowers. Keep your senses sharp.

Throughout your day, be conscious and connect with every activity that you do:

- Really smell and taste your food.
- Feel the cool leather of the easy chair underneath your skin. Feel your chair wrap around your body and nurture your body through your sense of touch and feeling,
- Listen to your environment. Really listen to the background noise in addition to the direct communication that is coming your way from the people in your life.
- Stimulate your emotion through music. Make music a more important part of your environment.
- Use fragrances to enhance your environment. Burn candles, potpourri, or cook with different spices.
- Feel your partner and let them feel you with both your sense of touch, and your heart. You will heighten your sense of feeling on every level when you truly connect this way. Sex is an exciting way to stimulate all your senses. How about that for an exciting 100 years!

When your five senses are fresh and on top of their game, your sixth sense will thrive. You will learn to trust your Innate, and you will follow your instincts toward your ideal 100 Year Lifestyle. At this stage in your life, your experience, combined with a heightening of your senses, will lead you down the right path. The top business leaders, athletes, and parents have all learned to trust their Innate. Keeping yourself fresh will heighten your senses and maximize the quality of your extended life.

CUSTOMIZE YOUR PERSONAL RENEWAL RECIPE

The purpose of your Personal Renewal Recipe is to help you stay fresh every day and make balance a part of your lifestyle. Balance is critical for your health and overall sense of wellbeing. When you venture out to tackle Your Next Big Thing, your Personal Renewal Recipe will be a healthy place to start from and come home to so you stay centered.

When you achieve balance inside your body, you will find that it is reflected outside of you as well. You will make better decisions professionally and personally, your relationships will improve, you may even find your finances take an upswing. All of a sudden, once-dormant areas of your life start to flourish. You may begin a hobby or sport that you have spoken about starting for years. Your efforts at work might start to receive more recognition. You may even find yourself making a lot of home improvements to enhance your environment. So many of us give so much of ourselves and wonder when it is going to come back. Your Personal Renewal Recipe will provide you with a permanent comes-back-to-you system that fills you up with the energy you want and need to continue to give your best you to the world.

Likewise, look back at times in your life when you were under a lot of stress. Maybe you had a lot of work pressures going on, or you were going through a relationship challenge. Despite your best efforts, can you see how your general state of internal disequilibria can filter into all aspects of life? You may have made poor relationship decisions, or jumped from one lousy work situation to another one. Rather than thriving, we downshift into survival mode when we are living out of balance. Resources feel scarce. You may find yourself being referred to as "selfish" or "self-centered" by others, and you may find yourself surrounded by a community of people desperate for things—grasping for love, money, or material possessions. This is a sign of your own internal state. Something in your life is stressing you and keeping you out of balance. Only you can determine the source and correct it. It may be a physical ailment, trouble in your marriage, financial problems, an untenable work situation, or even a housing situation that is no longer working for you.

Obviously you must do more than simply change your mind to change your life. You must make the changes by taking action. Your Personal Renewal Recipe can quiet the world and bring you back to center.

Can you see now why the most important relationship you will ever have, outside of your relationship with God, is with yourself, your Innate? You take yourself with you wherever you go.

While it is impossible to be perfectly balanced all the time, monitor your body and mind for balance, and make decisions to support that balance. You always want the pendulum to swing back to center. Your way back to "center" may include prayer or meditation, exercise, nutrition, meaningful work, family time, and personal time. Use the information you have learned so far to customize your plan. Your Personal Renewal Recipe will keep you in a state of balance that is aligned with your Innate Intelligence.

CUSTOMIZE YOUR PERSONAL RENEWAL RECIPE

Now it is time for you to design a Personal Renewal Recipe that you will rely upon to ensure that you start your day healthy, focused, and centered. It will reconnect you in the middle of the day to that same rock solid center, and help you finish your day there as well. The way that you start your day from this moment forward will determine the quality of your days and ultimately, the quality of your life.

FIRST HOUR: RENEWAL

What is the first thought, action, or feeling that you have when you start your day? Think about your first thought this morning immediately upon opening your eyes. Did you say to yourself, "I'm glad to be alive?" Or did you moan and groan?

A positive first thought, action, and feeling are important to get you on the right track. Ideal first thoughts might be, "I'm going to make today a great day." Another one might be, "I feel younger and healthier today." Another might be, "It feels good to be alive and I will embrace the day. I will create opportunities today where none exist. I will enjoy a relaxing time with my family today." Positive and happy thoughts have been shown to keep people feeling healthier and younger.

During that first hour, which you may find becomes your favorite part of the day, take the time to connect with your spiritual self through prayer, meditation, exercise, inspirational reading, stretching, goal setting or any other activity that gives you a feeling of renewal.

MIDDAY RENEWAL

When I was in private practice in Atlanta, Georgia, my practice got very busy. My office hours were 9 A.M. to 1 P.M. and 3 P.M. to 6 P.M. My patients used to laugh at me and joke with me about my two-hour lunch breaks. They would ask me, "What on earth are you doing for those two hours?"

While I would use some of this time for Prep work—writing reports, returning calls, and reading through some research—

I would also meditate or take a power nap during this time. This was essential to maintaining my own sense of renewal. My patients would pick up on that and were very supportive. After all, my days were spent working with over 100 patients per day who were either sick and suffering, or wanting to take their health to the next level. They needed me to be at the top of my game. This afternoon siesta made all the difference in the world for me and for them.

Centenarian Secret
Finding two hours to nap might not be possible for you, but we can all find 20 minutes to meditate on most days. Take the time. Make the time. Shut off your cell phone and e-mail devices and reconnect with your center for your midday renewal.

In many parts of the world, siestas are part of the culture. Everything closes down for two hours midday. Our bodies are not designed to be constantly "on" throughout the day. Siestas allow people to remain fresh—in the mornings and in the afternoons. Human beings need to recharge. Also, sitting on your tail for ten hours a day strains your spine, muscles, nervous system, and adrenal glands—it causes a tremendous amount of stress. This can lead to burnout in a hurry. Taking the midday break, meditating, going for a power walk, relaxing, and our minds and our bodies can keep you at the top of your game.

When you get off track with your daily renewal, remember Life Changing Principle Number 2 (Change happens one choice at a time—think progress, not perfection), and get back on track with your next choice.

NIGHT-TIME RENEWAL

This is a great time to spend with family and friends reading inspirational books and literature, reviewing your goals, reviewing the day, preparing for tomorrow, praying, or learning something new. Go to bed after you have tied up loose ends—this creates peace of mind and frees up your energy. Incomplete tasks can pile up and burden you through the night—lowering your energy and your capacity to embrace the opportunities and challenges of the day.

What would be the ideal way to end your days? Do you like to end your days with a workout, reading, listening to music or gathering with friends or family? To ensure your ideal 100 Year Lifestyle, it is important that you make choices for how you start and end your days.

Rock solid support comes from knowing how to support yourself, being willing to support others, and being involved with people. It is very important to invest your time in the people and relationships that are important to you. Lifelong learning can be a catalyst for steady growth and companionship. How do you balance it all with so much going on in your life? With Quality Time Living, of course, as you will see in the next chapter.

THE 100 YEAR LIFESTYLE
ACTION PLAN FOR LASTING CHANGE

1. Support yourself. Treat yourself the way you would want to be treated. Set an example for others. Apply the Three Life-Changing Principles to change the way you support yourself for an ideal 100 Years.

2. Commit to your Personal Renewal Recipe. Once you know what works for you, make it a priority. Make these things your Human Potential Pattern and a part of your lifestyle. Define your early-morning renewal, midday renewal, and nighttime renewal. Don't compromise.

3. Exchange support. Be willing to give the people you love and care about the kind of support that they need, even if it is different from the kind of support you like for yourself. Ask for the ideal support that you need from your life partner.

4. Establish Surround Sound Support. Expand your support system using the Health Care Hierarchy, multiple circles, and multiple generations. Build your awareness of the support system you desire and the people and resources that are already in your life. Plug the most important relationships into your Quality Time Calendar in the next chapter.

5. Balance your support system. If your current support system is great for crisis but empty for quality of life, joy, knowledge, and health, spend time building and nurturing support in these areas. Embrace multiple generations and multiple

circles of people. Step outside your current box. Make the time for the support you deserve.

6. Decide what you want to learn over the course of your 100 Year Lifestyle and take a first action step. Buy a book, enroll in a class or attend a seminar. Make an appointment with an expert. Choose a mentor. Create a long list, since you will have plenty of time to experience it all. Learning things you are passionate about will add passion to the rest of your life.

7. Trust your Innate Intelligence. Six Sense your life. Really begin to take notice and appreciate your surroundings with your vision, hearing, touch, taste, and smell, as well as your intuition. This will open you up to fresh ideas and ground you on the foundation upon which you wish to build your 100 Year Lifestyle.

PART 7

Quality Time Living: Making Every Moment Count

Whether you're working or whether you're playing, make it quality time.

CHAPTER 16

ACHIEVING THE ULTIMATE BALANCE OF TIME

Did you know that there are 525,600 minutes in a year? When I first did the math, I was blown away. Then I did the math for ten years. Do you realize that over the past ten years you've spent 5,256,000 minutes? Over the past twenty years you've had over 10 million minutes.

The number becomes nearly inconceivable when you understand that you may live over 100 years. If you reach your hundredth birthday, you will have lived a grand total of 52,560,000 minutes. That's a lot of minutes. The question, of course, is "Are you making the best use of the time?"

The Quality Time Living principles for The 100 Year Lifestyle will help you take your life to the next level and optimize every tick of your clock. The purpose of this Quality Time Living system is to fall madly in love with your life and give you control over how you spend your minutes. When you master the ability to make the most of your time, you will be very excited about the opportunities that lie ahead. You will get to the place where you love your Prime Time because you love your work and you love what you do. You will love Prep Time as well, because you love organizing yourself and planning for productive Prime Times and enjoyable Play Times. And you will love Play Time because you will be having more fun than you ever thought possible.

A NEW PERSPECTIVE ON TIME AS YOU AGE

When you are young and starting a job, you may not have as much control over how you spend your time—at least you think you don't. For the most part, you will be working for other people. You may have a young family. There are many demands on your time that may not be of your choosing. But as you mature and develop a little more financial stability, personal and professional confidence, you'll need to rethink the way you approach time. Time is both a tool and a resource. The good news is that there are more opportunities than ever to achieve the ultimate balance through the Quality Time Living strategies of The 100 Year Lifestyle.

There are many great opportunities in this new economy for people who are smart enough to see and capitalize on them. These days, the most financially successful people are not being paid by the hour, by the month, or even by the year. They are being paid for their talent and by the results they produce. In order to produce greater results for yourself, it will be helpful to change your strategy with respect to time. Time management is a very important component of The 100 Year Lifestyle.

There are examples everywhere of people who have not figured out how to capitalize on time. Recently, I was standing by my gate at the Las Vegas airport when a doctor approached me to discuss his practice. I had just finished up a seminar where he heard me speak. He told me that he was seven years into his practice and he had become a workaholic. He was financially successful but was driving himself into the ground—physically, emotionally, and spiritually.

His time wasn't his, and therefore neither was his life. He said that if he didn't make some changes, his life would come to a crashing halt. He sighed and said to me with despair, "If this is all there is, I don't want it."

We see this horrible imbalance very often today with two-income families who never get to see each other. They are working all the time and are typically all work and no play. They talk about business morning, noon, and night. They lose themselves in the process. Work is not simply a part of their life—work is their life. In my family practice I would see parents come in with their kids at all different times—trying to figure out a way to balance their busy schedules. In the process, they miss out on the quality time that they deserve as a family.

Centenarian Secret

Your minutes are your currency. They belong to you, and how you spend them will determine the quality of your life going forward. Every minute you spend represents a choice—whether you made it with full awareness or not. Take charge of your minutes.

Taking charge of how you spend your time ensures that you'll live a quality, purposeful life for the rest of your life. If you are ready to master time and capitalize on this wonderful opportunity, you can affirm your commitment by adding these words to your human potential pattern: "My minutes, my health, my life."

GET CONTROL OVER YOUR SCHEDULE

When you do what you love and enjoy your life, you experience a sense of timelessness. One hundred years will fly right by; yet, you will be present for every minute of it. If you are doing work that you love, have good health, and have a life filled with solid and loving relationships, you are very close to being there. But you must still change your perception of time to optimize the impact of your minutes. Otherwise, your life can easily devolve into any of the negative patterns we discussed in Part Two—with negative consequences such as divorce and ill health. Without the concepts and vision in place, and without the structure to achieve the balance, even under the best of circumstances, you will not optimize your 100 Year Lifestyle.

THE QUALITY TIME LIVING MODEL

To optimize your 100 Year Lifestyle, start by dividing your time into three different realms:

- Prime Time: This is about production. It is the time you designate to produce results, utilize your skills, and apply talents to generate value in the world. This is all about working in your professional life or for your favorite cause, and it is a very important part of staying sharp, purposeful, and productive.
- Prep Time: This is about organization and strategic planning. This is the time that you plan, organize, do research, and lay the groundwork for superb Prime Times and fabulous Play Times.
- Play Time: This is the free time you spend reading, getting massages, playing golf, doing yoga, traveling, going on hikes with your family, and taking vacations.

I remember when I first opened my training company, The Family Practice, and began teaching this time model to doctors. They were blown away by how much more focused they were with their patients. They started to take more vacations - Play Time - and found that adding this balance to their lives improved their personal relationships and made their life more fun.

The challenge for me was that our company grew so fast that I lost myself in the process and got off track with my own Prime Time, Prep Time, and Play Time. While I had mastered this time model in my practice, I had not yet figured out how to apply it to my new life. By disciplining myself to abide by my own Prime, Prep, and Play Time model, I was able to get back on track when I reconnected to "my life, my health, and my minutes."

When you run yourself ragged, just trying to keep up with the demands of your current job—and your present-day life—you are essentially treading water. Every day at work, you have the opportunity to learn new skills, sharpen existing skills, and gain new perspective on how to do things better. Unfortunately many of us aren't taking the time to process the information and get ahead of the game. We are always playing catch up. It's like we're eating a meal and then frantically moving on to the next meal without taking time to digest. We meet demand after demand, just hoping that one day things will magically get a little easier. When we see the signs of distress showing up in our lives, we often crash and say, "I need a vacation," and run that much faster until a crisis forces us to actually take one.

On a bigger scale, many of us do this until the age of 65, or whatever age at which we plan to retire. We go ballistic for 45 years of our working life and then come to a crashing halt in retirement. This "all or nothing' mentality and mindset can really burn us out, especially when our time is out of control. Quality Time Living will give you more control over your time than you have ever had before, and your choices will be driven by quality of life motivation.

HOW SUCCESSFUL PEOPLE REGARD TIME

You break out of this pattern by learning to look at your time very strategically.

Many highly successful people already use the time model we are going to discuss, even if they don't use the names Prime, Prep, and Play Time. Let's take, for example, one of my clients—a hip-hop and R & B performer and Grammy Award winner. I have seen him intermittently for many years as a chiropractic patient. When popular entertainers are on the road, which he often is, they often do different gigs in a different city every other night, sometimes every night. This can be a challenge.

They get through it by dividing up their time. When they are onstage performing before crowds, they are in Prime Time. When they are rehearsing, they are in Prep Time. And they incorporate downtime into their schedules as Play Time. In fact, I first met him at the beautiful spa Chateau Élan in Georgia while we were both relaxing on the couch, watching an NFL football game while waiting for a massage. We met while we were both enjoying our Play Time.

Entertainers like him make optimal use of their time—because they have to. They are peak performers and many people count on them. Most of us don't carry around quite this same level of responsibility. Nor do we have the benefit of people managing us and showing us how to make optimal use of our time. But knowledge is power and if you begin to value your talents and choose how you utilize your time with the same intention as these professionals, you will notice a giant step up in your quality of life on every level. Your Prime Times will quadruple in productivity, your Play Times will be much more fun and exciting, and you will stay organized through it all during Prep Time.

We've also heard stories of entertainers, athletes, and business-people who, because they don't understand the importance of this balance or don't have a structure to follow, are constantly in Prime Time and suddenly collapse—ending up in hospitals and suffering from stress and exhaustion. We see this with entrepreneurs who do the same. They go and go without giving their minds, bodies, and spirits the chance to revitalize and renew. Balance is crucial for creativity, sustained energy, and peace of mind. It's necessary for longevity. It's necessary for ongoing business success and the personal fulfillment of sharing this success with the most important people in your life and the philanthropic causes that feed your soul. This Quality Time Living model will give you the structure to truly have it all.

Remember Life Changing Principle Number 1: Change is easy. Thinking about change is hard. The reality of Quality Time Living is that you can rethink the way you look at the days, weeks, months, and years to reinvent your life and make the changes you know you need to make, without compromising your life. You can easily use this model to make your priorities *the* priority, even if you are currently locked into a "nine-to-five" job.

This is how you get off the treadmill and start building upon your time and experiences. One of my patients, Bruce Blythe, a very successful entrepreneur who owns the company Crisis Management International, understood this concept instinctively. He would travel and meet with companies to help them reach their goals, grow his business, and be productive during Prime Time. He would meet with his team when he was in town during Prime Time, and he would spend quality time at home or traveling the world with his family during Play Time. Like my clients, and many other successful people, he knows how to use his time for optimal results.

DON'T BE A TWENTY-FIRST-CENTURY TASKMASTER

When we feel like we have an endless amount of time to complete a task, we manage the task in a way to fill the time. If we have a month, we take a month, even if the project would require just a handful of focused days. Rather than letting our most important goals and significant results determine how we fill our days, many of us have become twenty-first-century taskmasters who are busy, busy, busy all the time but never seem to be getting anything done. This may be human nature for some of us, but not for the truly high achievers who want to be as productive as possible while also enjoying the most incredible Play Time in their lives. Become a Quality Time Living person and take yourself to the next level.

If I gave you 100 days in a row to get everything done that you needed to get done to organize your life, complete tasks that were weighing on you, clean up the messes you have laying around, work on your goals, and strategic plan for the next three years, could you be much more organized? Do you think you would get ahead of the game? Would you be able to formulate an action plan for your ideal 100 Year Lifestyle? Of course you could. You would love it because with 100 days you could put all the pieces in place to make things happen for the most productive Prime Times you've ever had, and the dream Play Times you've always wanted to take. If I gave you 300 days over the next three years, could you really, really set things up and get not just your current act together, but your second and third act as well? You wouldn't need that much time. You would be done so much quicker than you ever thought, because your time was focused.

The reality is that you would probably need only three quarters of this time, 75 days a year maximum, to set up your next three years exactly how you would like them to be. This is how you should think to make the best use of your Prep Time. Obviously the way our world is currently set up, you could not take these 75 days in a row, but you could scatter them throughout the year, designate them as Prep Time, and over the next year, two years, or three years make it happen. Are you starting to get the picture of how to use the Quality Time Living model? I've just given you those 75 Prep Time days a year or whatever number you think you would need based on your current life and your future goals. Your job is to think about your life and goals and decide on the number that would work for you. It's your 100 Year Lifestyle to live.

How much Prime Time do you need to double, triple, or even quadruple your income or production? If you had 100 intensely focused Prime Time days this year, would that be a good start? Would it take 150 days? What do you think would happen if you took these 150 days in a row? You would probably fry yourself with this constant intensity and burn yourself out. Is it any wonder that you feel exhausted all the time now if you feel like you have been living in constant Prime Time over the last 25 years? Think about how much more productive you could be, how much more money you would make, or how much more you could contribute if you took ownership over your time and focused your energy this way. What an energy enhancer it is to take control over your life with the structure of Quality Time Living.

Play Time is where it really gets fun. From this point forward, look at Play Time differently than you ever have before. You don't have to earn it, you don't have to be exhausted to take it, and you take as much of it as you can afford to take to enjoy the quality of life you deserve for 100 years and beyond. Can you imagine taking 365 Play Time days a year for the last 30 years of your life? This is complete retirement. The problem for many of today's retirees is that they get so out of balance with Play Time that it just isn't fun anymore. They get bored out of their mind without the balance of a productive purpose to keep them stimulated. How much Play Time would be enough to give you the balance you desire? What if you took 122 Play Time days a year and balanced it with the Prime Time and Prep Time to sustain you and keep you connected to your creative passions in the work world. If you truly enjoyed your vocation so that it also fed your soul while you continued to earn income, you would fill yourself up in all three aspects of Quality Time Living.

As your financial situation improves over time, you can balance your schedule with the number of Prime Time, Prep Time, and Play Time days to support your ideal 100 Year Lifestyle. Maybe you have had a great run and are financially independent but are tired of the 365 Play Time days a year and want to get back in the game. How many Prime, Prep, and Play Time days would get you engaged in your life again with the balance that would also keep your peace? What if you want to transition yourself to a new job or a new business? How many of each type of day would get you there? Step out of your Monday, Tuesday, Wednesday rut and begin to label your days, weeks, and months with this new model of time and watch how your results, contributions, and passions fill up your days. You will find yourself using this language and you will love it. Your friends and family members will love it too as you take them along for the ride. You will refine your quality of life as you age in years, rather than retiring into the grumpy old stage in which many of today's aging population have found themselves after being blindsided by their extended life.

We have become a nation of free agents. Our ability to continue to produce value throughout our 100 Year Lifestyle now lies in our creativity and experience—our ability to bring new ideas, thoughts, concepts, products, and results into the marketplace. In March 2006, *Fortune* magazine declared "innovation" as the "main competitive strength" in today's marketplace. This is why Quality Time Living is such a critical component of The 100 Year Lifestyle. This work-smart structure will help you adapt to this new paradigm.

PUTTING IT ALL TOGETHER

The way to manage your personal and professional lives in this new economy is to manage your schedule differently. Let's stop thinking we need to fit our life into our schedule and instead build our schedule around our life, talents, skills and passion. Stop thinking that one more sacrifice is going to yield the job security that you crave. It is not. You need to learn to work smart. This means managing your career around your life while you enjoy the balance. This will give you the upper hand—at work and in life.

> **Centenarian Secret**
>
> What happens when your life is out of balance?
>
> If you have too much Prime Time and not enough Prep and Play Time … you are probably reaching your professional goals but you are exhausted, your health is suffering, and you may be having challenges in your most important relationships, which can lead to resentment, pressure from home, or even divorce.
>
> If you have too much Prep Time and not enough Prime and Play Time … you are one of the busiest people you know but you never seem to be getting ahead financially, or have time to really connect to the people in your life.
>
> If you have too much Play Time and not enough Prime and Prep Time … you are either bored out of your mind and turning into a vegetable brain, or you are increasing your debt every year because you are not generating enough money to afford all of your play. Get back into balance with the Quality Time Living model.

If you are not building enough time into your life to play, try scheduling some real quality Play Time first. This is when great ideas are often born and when we begin to build our lives from a place of awareness.

Whenever you find yourself overwhelmed and "stuck" going forward, I want you to stop trying to address the problem by simply tacking on more Prime Time into your already too-busy schedule. You will generally find the solution you are looking for in Play Time. Step away for a day, a long weekend, or a week. You will not only find your solution, but you will also find yourself along with the natural energy to enjoy your life.

FOCUSING YOUR TIME

You will love what happens when you begin to prioritize the "Play Time" component of your schedule—and actually begin to build your schedule around it. Start to make your life as important, or more important, than your work. You can set up your life to have a blast. As the quality of your Play Time improves you will find yourself more focused than ever during your Prime Times and your Prep Times because you know you have terrific Play Time coming down the pike. This triune of time will help you create the balance to optimize every phase of your life.

Play Time keeps life fun, exciting, and balanced. I first discovered this system in the early 1990's when I was busy with my practice, trying to provide the optimum care to my patients, without compromising the quality of life with my family. I had lofty goals for my chiropractic practice and patients, but I also wanted to coach my kids in T-ball and soccer teams.

I found that thinking of the regular workweek as "just another Monday" and TGIF (thank God it's Friday) just didn't work to create the level of success and balance that I wanted. However, I did find that when I focused my time when I was with patients—the same way that a professional athlete, entertainer, or neurosurgeon focuses on his or her craft—my success with patients rose dramatically, along with my patient volume.

This was very exciting, but then I ran into problems when I kept this intensity all the time. It caused a lot of problems in my marriage and kept me from being present with my children. It was out of the need to find this balance for myself that I learned to follow this system. I then refined it as I began traveling and teaching other doctors and business leaders about this model.

I have consulted with over thousands of doctors who have also benefited from Quality Time Living. Many physicians struggle mightily with this issue. For many of them, they start off incredibly imbalanced time-wise as young adults because of the rigor of their training. And once they are finished, they are left with the burden of building a practice during the very same years that many of them are starting families. I have seen many people watch their relationships falter under the burden of this stress. You don't have to experience these challenges anymore. Isn't it exciting to know you can take more time off and increase your production dramatically, both at the same time?

TIME MANAGEMENT AND THE 100 YEAR LIFESTYLE

How will knowing that you'll probably live longer than you ever imagined affect the way you view time? At first I thought it might cause people to procrastinate. I thought they'd say, "Why bother? I have plenty of time?" But just the opposite has been true. In fact, I have found that one of the reasons people procrastinate is that they say to themselves, "Why bother? I won't have enough time to complete what I start." Or, "Why bother? I don't have the time to acquire new skills or enjoy the fruits of my labor."

Your awareness of extended living will motivate you to pursue your dreams, knowing you will have all the time you need to make the most of them. Procrastination can be a source of incredible suffering. I have seen numerous patients put off the inevitable chiropractic care that they needed, only to require much more intensive, more expensive care down the road because they waited too long. To make matters worse, they are left with more residual damage in their spine, nervous system and entire body.

I recently reviewed a spinal x-ray of a man in his fifties who finally decided to come in for a chiropractic checkup alleviate and take action on his health. I showed him his x-rays in two parts. We compared his healthy bones and joints with his damaged ones. I asked him how old his healthy bones looked. He said they looked around 30 years old. When he looked at the bones in his neck, he sadly said to me, "Those bones look like they are 80 years old." Obviously all of his bones are the same age. However, each part of your body ages differently based on how it is aligned and balanced. Procrastination has drastic effects on your body.

Procrastination can also cause suffering when you know you're capable of accomplishing more with your talents. Knowing that you are not living up to your capabilities can be a real blow to your self-esteem.

Many of us have spent the first 30 or 40 years scattering energy all over the place because of our inability to focus our time. We don't target it. We try to be all things to all people, even as our confidence and self-esteem slide lower and lower or our health starts to slip. This is a game you simply can't win. Build a life of integrity by prioritizing and focusing your energy on the things that matter to you and set yourself up to win for the rest of your life by choosing the way you spend your minutes.

Time is one of your greatest assets as you live your ideal 100 Year Lifestyle.

CHAPTER 17

PRIME TIME, PREP TIME, AND PLAY TIME: AN EXCITING, FRESH MODEL OF TIME

Let's look at this time model in greater depth and apply it to your life. The Quality Time Living model of The 100 Year Lifestyle will show you how to balance your life to optimize your financial, professional, and personal fulfillment. The first thing you need to do is to look at your weeks, months, and years as something greater than simply Sunday, Monday, Tuesday, Wednesday, Thursday, Friday, and Saturday. From now on, begin to think of these days as Prime Time, Prep Time, and Play Time.

As you understand and master this new way of looking at time, you'll discover some exciting things. You will get more done in less time than you thought possible. You'll find that your Play Time increases in quality. You will get the rest and rejuvenation that you need and the travel and adventure you want. You'll become more organized as you plant the seeds for the ultimate Prime Time and the ultimate Play Time.

If you have never looked at time this way before, you haven't really had ownership over your days, your weeks, your months, and your years. Haven't we all heard of individuals who neared burnout and then decided to step back and spend less time at work, and then they really struck it rich? The reason is because when you live in balance, your energy goes directly toward your creativity. When you are constantly exhausted and stressed, your energy goes toward survival—it goes toward managing the stress inside your body and pushing you through fatigue.

If you are self-employed, I really recommend that you allot days specifically for Prime, Prep, and Play Time. That is not to say they will be 100 percent devoted to one thing or another. You may spend 80 to 90 percent of your day in Prime Time on a Prime Time day, for example, and then 20 percent on Prep Time. But in general, you want to make it a complete Prime Time, result-oriented day. If you are working in a job in which you don't have as much control, try to set up your schedule so that your Prime Time matches your supervisor's or company's Prime Time.

PRIME TIME

Prime Time days are about generating results, building relationships, or generating money—to use your talents and abilities in ever more effective ways to create more value in the world. That value will generate the money to finance your 100 Year Lifestyle. But don't do things just for the money. Do things you love to do and formulate them into a business model that finances your 100 Year Lifestyle.

As you generate money, decide in your Prep Time where to invest it, so you can move your life in the direction that you desire. Also, the quality of your Prep Times will have a tremendous impact on the quality of your Prime Time and Play Time.

Here are some examples in different professions:

Teacher: Let's say you are a teacher. Your Prime Times are when you teach classes. Your Prep Times are for organizing, grading tests, and creating lesson plans.

Writer: If you are a writer, your Prime Times are spent writing. Prep Time is spent on research.

Salesperson: For a salesperson, Prime Time is spent in front of customers and potential customers. Prep Time is spent on getting ready to spend time with customers, and on organization, reviewing sales numbers, and setting goals.

CEO: If you are a CEO, your Prime Time may be spent meeting with your board, shareholders, or key customers. Your Prep Time is spent on planning, delegating to staff, and constructing the future of your company.

Athlete: If you are an athlete, your Prime Time is the day of the game. Prep Time is spent practicing on the field or working out in the gym.

Manager: If you are a manager, Prime Time is when you are meeting with your team to ensure their productivity. Prep Time may be spent setting goals, organizing, or researching a new business system.

Entertainer: If you are an entertainer, Prime Time is the time you spend on the stage or on the television show or movie set. Your Prep Time is spent on rehearsals, makeup, and reading scripts.

In any of these examples, if you don't spend enough time on your Prep Times, the quality of your Prime Times will be reduced. If you are a musician and you didn't spend enough time on rehearsal, for example, you probably won't deliver a good performance. Prime Time isn't only about execution, however. It is also the time when we utilize our talents. My wife, Lisa, for example, is an incredible photographer and artist. Over the years she nurtured her photographic eye and her passion for art, design, and technology. For the longest time she wasn't sure where her journey would take her. All of a sudden things came together. Now, during her Prime Times she has an opportunity to do what she loves—making multimedia masterpieces for herself and our company. Her Prime Time is taking photography courses and on the computer creating masterpieces. Her Prep Time is spent doing research. You can apply this model of time no matter what you do.

If you fully embrace this model of time, it will radically change your life. One of my clients in Australia recently said to me that after implementing Quality Time Living, he cut his hours from five and a half days a week to three and a half and he focused and improved the quality of the care he provides dramatically while increasing his practice by $360,000 a year. I told him in a joking manner that he should consider going to two days a week.

My yardman listened to some of the audio CDs that I made on this topic and quadrupled his business in two years. You can do the same, and you will have a blast in the process.

On the other hand, another one of my new clients came to see me a while back. He was burned out. I asked him, "When was the last time you took a vacation?" He said, "It's been ten years." When I asked him how his wife felt about that, he told me he had just gone through a divorce. This is what happens when people spend too much time in Prime Time. This is a classic, "all work and no play" scenario. It's very draining and leads to fatigue, ill health, being overweight, and broken relationships. Stay in Prime Time for too long and eventually you can expect some sort of health or relationship crisis to come your way.

For the rest of your life, I would like you to make Play Time a priority in your lifestyle. You don't have to earn it, prove yourself, or put it off until next year. You deserve it, and Play Time will come first when you schedule it into your life. So many of us run ourselves into the ground and collapse at the finish line so we can get away for a weeklong vacation, and then go back to work and do it again. Finding the perfect balance of Prime, Prep, and Play Time is essential for ensuring a quality of life as you age. When you schedule your life this way, you choose your focus and build momentum.

PREP TIME

Prep Time is about organization. It is about preparing for great Prime Times and Play Times. The trick with Prep Time is that you may not see the results of your work right away because you are laying down the tracks. This is where the discipline comes in to work on your life and business, rather than just be caught up in it. For example, think of a beautiful garden in the summer. When you look around, you see flowers in bloom—red, yellow, pink, and white blossoms. They are fragrant. A butterfly lands on a cluster of strawberries and spreads its wings. The garden is in full bloom, showing its magnificent beauty and producing a sense of abundance.

The days that you are sitting in the garden and enjoying it with your family are Play Time days. Planning the garden to begin with took place during Prep Time. Building the garden was the Prime Time activity. Utilize this triune of time properly and you truly find the balance you can enjoy for a lifetime.

> ### Centenarian Secret
> Have you ever felt like your days were a hodgepodge of Prime, Prep, and Play blended together? When this happens you will find that you get half as much done in twice the time with quadruple the stress. Quality Time Living is a much better option.

Fulfilled, successful people are masters of time. They know that when they set things up the right way, the right things happen. For them, their Prep Times are spent on developing their business model, marketing, networking, doing interviews, setting goals, researching new technology, and participating in panel discussions. They work on building and nurturing relationships that support their primary purpose. It can take weeks, months, or even years, in some cases, to see the full fruit of their Prep Time efforts but when they do the right things, for the right reasons, they can expect to eventually reap the right results. This is the magic of Prep Time.

The risk of Prep Time is spending too much time on the "doing" without generating production in Prime Time. Think about the real estate investor who looks and looks but never buys—or the doctoral candidate who works on his thesis for years but fails to present. Prep Time, for some, becomes a way to avoid risk. This is the "Constantly Busy but Not Accomplishing Anything" syndrome. For example, I had a client who was very hard to get on the phone. He always seemed to be busy. In fact, he was one of the busiest guys I'd ever seen. Unfortunately for him, his practice wasn't getting him anywhere but in a state of exhaustion. He never seemed to be able to get over the hump. Eventually, you need to pull the trigger and do the things that generate results.

PLAY TIME

Play Time is simply about enjoying your life. On a Play Time day, you are not busy trying to stay organized. You are doing whatever it is that makes you happy and rejuvenates you—reading a good book at home or on the beach, going for a walk in the woods, spending time with your life partner, traveling to exotic places, and celebrating life. When you look at your schedule for the next 12 months, what I would like you to do is to start blocking off your Play Time days first. This might seem counterintuitive to what you have always done. Play Time first is a key component of The 100 Year Lifestyle. Play Time days, however, aren't only for rest and relaxation.

Play Time will cultivate your creativity. Your creativity is ultimately the force behind the exciting and passionate 100 Year Lifestyle you want to enjoy. It will not only be what gets you ahead in this new era, but it will also help you choose new and exciting goals and adventures that you'd like to experience. I'm sure you know there are a million forces at work to ensure you don't take the time to nurture this creativity. The tendency, today, is to push and push—to keep working day and night and to stay plugged in. Scheduling Play Time first is about setting boundaries. It is also showing the world, and yourself, that you value your life and your family, and you do so by making them your first priority.

Centenarian Secret
Play Time frees up your creativity, creates balance, and frees you from the grind and the intensity of Prime Time. Play Time frees up your energy, relaxes you, balances out your system, and produces a condition of homeostasis–a condition of equilibrium–throughout your mind and body. It is often where Your Next Big Thing is born.

Many people report that their creativity comes out in Play Time, which is another reason why you need to take it. What's interesting is that when many of us are in a rut, we try to work ourselves out of it and instead we just end up digging it deeper. The way to get out of a rut is to step away and take Play Time. Life is not just about work. You deserve to enjoy your life. Have fun and lots of it. In fact, since you are going to have more time than you originally thought you would, why not have more fun than you ever dreamed possible.

Schedule "Play Time" days around important birthdays, anniversaries, Valentine's Day, and other holidays, including Memorial Day and Labor Day. And then if you know you are going to take specific vacations, mark those off as well. The next step, after recording all of your key Play Time days, is to record your key Prime Time days.

When people retire or settle into Play Time too much, they risk falling into a complacency or comfort pattern. Once again, the key here is balance. When you are young and working, you may need to be reminded to include Play Time in your overall life planning. Maybe you have played too much in relation to how much Prime Time you have taken and you have no money. Your balance may need to shift back in the Prime Time direction. However, as you gain experience and financial independence, schedule enough Prime Time to fulfill your passions and commitments, and to reach your goals. But just know that all play and no work can lead to vegetable brain, negativity, and increasing debt or using up your assets. If you have no purpose and you are drifting, it can take its toll on your passion for life.

This is why complete retirement has become a problem for many retirees. I know a doctor who had been in practice for 60 years. In 60 years he had rarely missed a day at work and was almost never sick. As soon as he retired, he found that he had way too much time on his hands. He didn't pick up a hobby or cause to get behind, and he found it hard to engage in his life. He developed numerous health problems and became very stressed out. When he heard me speak about this topic he decided to go back into practice for two days a week. It was a great balance for him and amazingly, his retirement ailments cleared up.

CREATING YOUR PERSONAL QUALITY TIME CALENDAR

When you plan to achieve balance, you are connecting to what is really important to you. When you are young in your career, you might work five days a week and a half day on Saturdays, leaving only Sundays for true Play Time days. If you took every Sunday off for a year, plus two weeks' vacation, then you would have had 52 Sundays plus 14 Play Time days, or 66 Play Time days that year. As time goes on and you get better at mastering production, you might take every weekend off, which is 104 Play Time days—plus two weeks of vacation—which totals 118 Play Time days for the year. When you achieve financial independence and freedom, you may choose 200 Play Time days with 75 Prime Time and 90 Prep Time days. It's your calendar, your life, and your goals. You get to choose.

Get yourself a yearlong calendar and three different color markers. Designate one for Prime Time, one for Prep Time, and one for Play Time. Start with Play Time, and mark Play Time days for the year. Include all holidays, plus important birthdays, anniversaries, and school breaks if you have kids or grandchildren.

Next, block in all of your key Prime Time days. This would include big shows or conferences that are key generators of income in your industry or a cause in which you are involved. Include speaking engagements or seminars you want to attend—which may fall on weekends. Once this is done, block out every other "leftover" weekend as Play Time.

Next, block out the full weeks of vacation that you want to take. You might do this around school breaks—including the winter and spring holiday sessions, Presidents' Day weekend, and any other extended times when school is closed. You may choose to schedule them over Memorial and Labor Day weekends and Fourth of July.

As your children grow and begin their own families, you might choose to schedule one of your weeks to coincide with your children's and grandchildren's time off so you can enjoy this quality time with them. If you want to avoid the crowds, you may choose to avoid these holidays and go during the off-season.

Once your Play Time is blocked out, fill in your Prep Time and Prime Time throughout the weeks to support your ideal production and planning schedule. It may take you some time to develop the routine that supports your optimum production, efficiency, organization, health, and energy levels. You may find that taking a solid week of business travel works for your health, family, and energy. And then you might schedule the next several days as Play Time. Maybe you like one month on and one month off. As you move along in your career, you might even do one year on and one year off. The beauty of this plan is that it is extremely flexible. You cultivate a schedule to match your talents, goals, and the vision you have for your life.

YOUR QUALITY TIME CALENDAR AND YOUR 100 YEAR LIFESTYLE

Your ratio of Prime, Prep, and Play Time days will vary as you grow in income, security, and age. When you are in your twenties and thirties, you may find a ratio of 200 Prime Time days, 100 Prep Time days, and 65 Play Time days works for you. When you are in your forties and fifties and more secure, you may choose 150 Prime Time days, 50 Prep Time days, and 165 Play Time days. There is no rule as to how many of each you choose and you can vary the schedule as your financial life improves and you reach different goals. It's your year, it's your life, and you get to choose your own Quality Time Calendar.

Plan your schedule the way you want. Build flexibility into your plan. When you plan out your life this way, you can build rhythm into your plan and gain momentum for your career and your Play Time. Connect your calendar to your Personal Renewal Recipe and master your energy. When things are random, you have probably found that you never seem to get things rolling or off the ground. You are easily derailed from your objectives. It is easy to lose focus.

After a few months you will really get the hang of this planning strategy. You and your friends, family members, and coworkers will find yourselves using this new language and saying things like, "I'm in Prime Time tomorrow," or "today is Prep Time." Not only is it productive, but it will also help you understand each other and give the people in your life the support they need.

YOUR NEXT 30 DAYS

The important thing to understand, here, is that how you spend your time is one of the key things over which you have control—that will directly impact the quality of your 100 Year Lifestyle. These are your 52 million minutes; how are you going to choose to spend them? Now, I know that you are busy. I know that you are a responsible person, living an active life. I know that you are probably thinking right now of a hundred reasons why you can't change the way you view and manage time. Starting today, begin working on thinking of a hundred reasons why you can and get really excited about your life. Operate with faith that if you take the leap into your ideal 100 Year Lifestyle, and start doing things for the right reasons, you will love your life because you love the way you spend your time.

If planning the next year seems like too big of a leap right now, start with the next 30 days. Write down the most important Play Time and Prime Time goals that you have over the next month. If there are any fixed dates that you cannot change, enter them on the calendar accordingly. Decide how many Prep Time days you will need to be your best during those days and block them out. Fill in the rest of those 30 days to support your optimum Prime Time production and Play Time enjoyment.

Watch your energy, your professional production, and your personal fulfillment begin to soar. Get excited about the opportunities to have more fun than ever and generate more income than ever as you move to the next chapter and finance your incredible 100 Year Lifestyle.

THE 100 YEAR LIFESTYLE
ACTION PLAN FOR LASTING CHANGE

1. Get a yearlong calendar that also has a month at a glance. Decide on your most important Prime Time, Prep Time, and Play Time goals over the next 30 days. Fill in your Play Time days first and label them "Play Time" using a colored pencil. Then, in another color, indicate your most important Prime Time days that are already prescheduled.

2. Look at your goals and think through how many Prime Time days it will take you to reach your goals. Strategically color-code them on your calendar.

3. Determine how many Prep Time days it will take you to organize yourself to make your Prime Times a record-setting experience and at the same time, make your Play Time more enjoyable than ever.

4. Fill in the rest of your calendar with Prime Time, Prep Time, and Play Time days that will support you in reaching your goals.

5. Stay focused on each day, being true to its designated purpose, allowing for minor overlaps of activities since you are new to this system. Mastering this system is a process that takes time and you should remember the Three Life-Changing Principles throughout the process and keep your ideal 100 Year Lifestyle in mind.

6. Set up your entire year following the same guidelines. Build flexibility into your schedule and watch your productivity and passion soar as you achieve the ultimate balance.

7. Protect your time. Make your Play Times as fun and relaxing as possible, make your Prime Times as fun and productive as possible, and use your Prep Time to keep your life organized to optimize your Play Times and Prime Times. Have more fun than ever, making the most of your minutes.

PART 8

Financing Your 100 Year Lifestyle

Package your passion and attract money for a lifetime.

CHAPTER 18

YOU'RE GOING TO NEED MORE THAN YOU THOUGHT

The 100 Year Lifestyle is the greatest financial opportunity that we could ever imagine for us individually, and as a society. As you know, a key element of The 100 Year Lifestyle is taking care of your health, so you can optimize your quality of life and enjoy longevity. But because of that, you also have the opportunity to remain productive, well into your later years, generate more money than you ever dreamed of, and contribute more back to the world.

YOU'RE GOING TO NEED MORE THAN YOU THOUGHT FOR LONGER THAN YOU THOUGHT

So, what does remaining productive look like? For Jack Cashin, it's a polo field in Georgia named Chukkar Farm and Polo Club. He hosts polo matches for large gatherings and also runs a horse camp, gives riding lessons, and rides himself daily—at the time of this writing he was in his 80s. He also continues to play in polo matches himself. He has combined his love of horses with his love of the land, and he has continued to generate money into his eighth decade of life. He is a prime example of someone living The 100 Year Lifestyle.

He has led a fascinating life, comprised of myriad chapters—he bought an island in the Bahamas, ran for governor, founded and operated a chain of restaurants, and he has modeled for magazines and played polo with a prince. We are going to talk a lot in this chapter about the myriad "acts" that make up a life. This is a new phenomenon we are now seeing in response to the population's greater longevity, and a new economy. Surveys show that the majority of people over 60 intend to continue to generate money and value in the marketplace. They plan to continue working either full- or part-time, as consultants or by setting up their own companies. In some cases, they have logged many years at a corporation or in a single profession and are beginning their "Second Acts"—pursuing a career that may be more fulfilling and flexible. In other cases, they may have pursued a variety of paths throughout their lives and are now on their third, fourth, or fifth acts.

Even though the recent recession has presented challenges to many, we are still living in exciting financial times. Shift your perspective from thinking that financing a terrific 100 Year Lifestyle is going to be hard, or that if you live to be 100 you may run out of money. Instead, get excited about the opportunities and all the possibilities that exist in the next phase of your financial life and embrace them. You have the time to pursue a multitude of passions, paths, and interests and live your dream life financially.

Retirement is quickly becoming an outdated concept. *The Merriam-Webster Dictionary* defines it as "to go away, retreat, or withdraw." It was a concept that was created for world where the average life expectancy was 60 to 65 years. The plan was to work for a company for 30 to 40 years, retire, and then go away, retreat, or withdraw from society until you die just a few years later. Is this your plan for your extended life, knowing that you may have 35 years left? How many years of a purposeless life will it take to turn your mind into mush?

Many of today's young adults are learning about the changes to retirement from their older generations and are planning for the future differently. Using the Quality Time Living model and combining the balance of meaningful Prime Times, Prep Times and Play Times is a way to refine the next phase of your life. Instead of *retirement*, how about we think of the term *refinement*? This next phase of your life should be about refining and mastering your lifestyle. You should be able to move with ease between your Prime, Prep and Play Times and define how you spend your time so you are having a blast, making a difference, and optimizing the use of your talents and creativity while also increasing income. That is ideal. Boomers who have been surveyed on their retirement views say they want a "flexible" work arrangement that allows them to work intensely for shorter periods of time, with maximum production and minimal effort, while enjoying life to the fullest with as much Play Time as possible. Again, this is the concept of Quality Time that we've been discussing throughout this book, and it will help you to finance your ideal 100 Year Lifestyle.

Centenarian Secret

This desire for a flexible work schedule is very common for today's retirees as more, and more of them are going back to work. Some key reasons that retirees want to continue to work, aside from generating more money, include a desire to stay mentally active, a desire to stay physically active, and a desire to remain productive or useful.

RETHINKING "RETIREMENT"

With all the opportunities that exist, why live off of your portfolio as early as your mid-sixties? If you wait to claim Social Security until you are 70, 80, 90 years of age or older, you will get higher benefits than you would at 65 while continuing to have purpose and utilizing your talents to the fullest. That's just one benefit. But why not also use the passions and expertise that you have accumulated over the years to build and supplement your income, stimulate your mind, and give you purpose throughout your extended life? These are important options and choices that you'll want to consider as you question whether or not you really want to retire, especially when you have the realization that through Quality Time Living you can take as much Play Time as you want. Choosing to work is a world away from having to work. It is the difference between doing what you love vs. feeling trapped by your circumstances.

> Retire in Practice -Dr. Jay and Kathi Handt
> "There are a finite number of hours in every day, so you have to decide how you are going to use those hours for maximum enjoyment, enrichment, connection and prosperity. The aim is to prosper so you may live well and love everything you do."

This is a key reason why investing in yourself, your education and your passion throughout your life is so important. Joseph Cowen, for example, ran a successful business with his wife, Marie, for 30 years. They had initially discovered clay on their property and, as a result, started Sheffield Pottery. Cowen spun the pots and his wife designed the pottery. They grew that company to become one of the largest suppliers of ceramic supplies and retail pottery in the East, and their youngest son, John, runs that business today.

In his early sixties, Cowen started to look for a way to retire from pottery, in part to care for his ailing spouse. He began to invest in real estate. He eventually turned real estate into his second career after he discovered that he had a tremendous knack for it. He learned from his father, Jack Cowen, who was great real estate investor also. "When you buy, you sell" he would say in his beautiful Irish brogue—meaning that the gains are always in buying at the right price. For over 20 years, he has run his own real estate business and at age 85, he had 15 rental houses and two apartment buildings, which he actively manages.

If you approach your 100 Year Lifestyle from this perspective, you can also enjoy and extend your Prime earning years. You don't want to slave away at a job that you hate for 40 years in order to save for retirement. If you do, you can pretty much bank on your retirement being lousy too. This is not the balance we are looking for here. Don't work yourself so hard that you end up losing your health along the way. In my practice I saw so many patients who lost their health trying to accumulate wealth in the first 50 years of their life, only to spend their wealth to try and get their health back in their extended life. You will have to pay a heavy price to get it back once it is lost. Achieving the right balance is what The 100 Year Lifestyle is really all about.

Living The 100 Year Lifestyle:
On My First 100 Years by Joseph Angelo Enea

As of November 4, 2004, I am over 100 years old—that's a lot of presidents and macaroni!

Someone asked me about 25 years ago, "Mr. Enea, what is the secret to your longevity?" I replied, "Buying Certificates of Deposit that mature in 20 years." On my 92nd birthday, my son had a surprise party for me. As a joke, in front of all the guests, he made out a birthday check for $10,000.00, but dated it November 4, 2004—my hundredth birthday. Ever since then, I've reminded him to have the money ready. As a matter of fact, I had it framed and hung it in the living room of my house. Needless to say, when my son came to visit two days before the big event, November 2, 2004, the first thing I said was, "Did you bring the money?"

About ten years ago, I informed my son in a very serious tone, "Well son, I finally got the lots." He thought I meant cemetery lots. After a few seconds of more thought, he said, "Pop, you bought the two burial lots next to Grandma's and Grandpa's grave in Frankfort, New York." Flabbergasted, I replied, "What cemetery lots? No! I bought the two lots in back of our house that that bastard Tom Morreallo refused to sell me 20 years ago! I bought them from his son, who sold them to me for the price that his father refused to accept before he died." It pays to be patient.

Speaking of cemetery lots, I finally did get them in Frankfort. My son asked me, "Dad, how much did you pay for the lots?" "Cheap! I got them for nothing," I told him. He then asked, "How?" I said, "Well, since Uncle George Congilero is buried in Phoenix and Uncle Johnny in California, Aunt Gracie decided to give your mother and me the two lots that were reserved for them, next to Grandma and Grandpa Congilero."

"Even in death," my son said, "you've got an angel."

If you're wondering, dear reader, about that $10,000.00 check, here's what happened. At my hundredth birthday party at Grimaldi's Restaurant in Utica, in front of all my relations, my son made good on that check. He paid me $10,000, in ten $1,000 bills. The only problem was that the bills were in Italian lire, worth about $8.98, total, in American money. What's the difference? American, Italian? Who cares? We all had a good laugh.

Second, third, and even fourth acts are a critical component of keeping the passion flame burning for the balance of your 100 Year Lifestyle. Often they are even more splendid than first acts. Many boomers are starting new businesses in place of their retirements.

Your Prep Time and Play Time are the times to begin exploring your exciting, new ideas.

THE NOTION OF "FINANCIAL FREEDOM" INSTEAD OF RETIREMENT

As you have seen throughout this book, planning your life with an eye on the future will spare you much hardship. Robert Sullivan, a certified financial planner in Los Altos, California, says that views on retirement and retirement planning have changed greatly over the three decades he's been in the business. The focus now isn't on saving for retirement as much as it is on working toward financial freedom.

"This allows us to orient the decision-making process toward a time in our lives when we will be free to make choices and be less encumbered by the imperative to pay the bills. Our goal is to start liberating ourselves from "job and career" so we can enjoy life more now, perhaps even feel "rich" right where we are, without living a life of drudgery that ends someday in retirement."

"My dad was a great example. He worked two jobs most of his life — one in corporate management, and he owned a small machine shop. After I graduated from college and started my career in 1978, he dutifully became one of my first clients. I diligently went about trying to ascertain my dad's retirement goals and he skillfully dodged me for many years. He was enjoying his work so much it didn't make a lot of sense to him to be so focused on retirement. But he liked the idea of financial independence — having choices, control over his life, and choosing how he spent his time. This means control of the calendar."

THE FINANCIAL GIFT OF YOUR EXTENDED LIFE

By this stage in your life, you are probably in one of three positions financially:

1. You've hit the big time and reached your financial goals. You have all the money you'll ever want or need. You have accu-

mulated assets that will finance your present and future, and you are in superb financial condition. For you this book was more about health, relationships, how you spend your time, and your legacy. You are less concerned about re-evaluating your asset allocation, estate, and financial legacy, as you already have a team in place to help you continue to meet your goals. You meet with them regularly to discuss your goals — for today and tomorrow.

2. Second, you might be on your way toward reaching your goals. You have a good income stream and have begun to accumulate cash generating assets while paying down your debts. You invest in yourself regularly. Stay on your path. Look to use your skills and talents to create multiple income streams. Speak to your financial advisor, insurance agent, and estate planner, and re-evaluate your plan for your longevity. Discuss your plan with your life partner. If you haven't reached all your financial goals yet, don't worry! You have more time than you thought to get in excellent financial condition. It requires focus, discipline, and consistency. If your goal is to become a millionaire, which is not as much money as it used to be, you might want to place a "multi" in front of it, lay out the path, and enjoy the journey.

3. Third, you might be in financial trouble. If this is the case, you've got to make learning about money a priority. You are going to have plenty of time to master money, so you may as well begin to make managing it effectively a priority. Check your credit score and learn what it means. Meet with a financial planner and commit to a plan. You have got to change your relationship with money. Not changing will just perpetuate your financial suffering. Remember, change is easy;

thinking about change is hard. There is only one thing worse than financial suffering, and that is suffering for 100 years.

CHANGING YOUR FINANCIAL FOCUS

When it comes to investing in your future, set benchmarks and make your financial freedom a priority. Do you have a plan that is current? Is it real and based on your present financial position? Was it a plan that you put in place years ago that is in radical need of an update? Start investing now. Invest in yourself first. Invest in your education. Invest in your ideal 100 Year Lifestyle.

Many of today's teens and 20-somethings are already starting to invest in themselves. This happened in direct response to the nation's concerns about Social Security. As opposed to sticking their heads in the sand, they are arguably savvier about money than any generation before. The problem for many of us is that we take a short-term approach to money that is based on a 60-year lifestyle rather than a 100 Year Life-style. We can only see what we need today. Readjust your thinking and open your eyes to the fact that what is good for you in the long-term is also good for you today. Can you imagine going through your 30s, 40s, and 50s knowing that your independence is essentially already taken care of because you invested in yourself throughout your lifetime?

What's great about embracing your longevity is that even if you wait until you're in your 40s or 50s to start, you still have time to turn your financial life around and secure your future. Don't procrastinate; work your plan and get excited about it. Your best is yet to come. You can still live your dream while enjoying the balance of Quality Time Living.

REFINING YOUR WAY THROUGH RETIREMENT

The good news is that a sizeable portfolio is not your only option for a happy retirement. You will probably end up generating revenue for many more years than you originally thought since you will be refining yourself rather than retiring. Many of the current generation of 50-, 60-, and 70-year-old workers look to retirement so they can stop being miserable in their unfulfilling jobs. This is not The 100 Year Lifestyle. Do what you love with passion so you never get tired. Do what you love and you will attract lots of money. So regardless of your current position, you should still have plenty of time to reach your financial goals. Still, this is not an excuse to procrastinate. You must start investing in yourself today, if you haven't started already.

The sooner you start investing in yourself, the more time your money will have to grow. Put time on your side. Make investing a high priority. Create a plan, stick to it, and set goals for yourself. Remember, it's never too early or too late to start investing so start now, whatever your age!

Centenarian Secret
You Can't Afford to Get Sick!
Many people are concerned that they cannot afford healthy lifestyle choices such as buying organic foods, exercising, chiropractic adjustments, or an occasional massage. You absolutely can afford these and should make them a priority. Do you want to know what you can't afford? Here's what you can't afford: You cannot afford to get sick! Watch The 100 Year Lifestyle YouTube video, "You Can't Afford to Get Sick!"

CHAPTER 19

CAPITALIZING ON YOUR PAST TO CREATE CAPITAL FOR YOUR FUTURE

Your past has taught you a lot about money. What you learned about money in the past affects how you make, spend, and handle it today, so examine your beliefs and your results. Are your current financial beliefs and habits taking you toward your goals?

The truth is that most things in life come with a price tag. This includes the basics like shelter, water, food, heating, and cooling—everything. Take long-term planning into account with respect to your money and invest your funds wisely, or you will be caught up in a survival pattern. Think about how you have earned money up until now. Think about where you have spent money in the past. Many people get caught up in "competitive" spending. They try to keep up with the Joneses—at home and at work. Have you ever engaged in a game of one-upmanship with coworkers, friends, or neighbors? What was it like when the job was over? Or when the Joneses moved away? Did you ever wish you had passed on the new car or the latest gadgetry and invested more in the things that matter to you? What would you do differently now?

Capitalize on your past to create capital for your future. I've certainly made mistakes in the past. But those mistakes made it possible for me to achieve greater financial success, just as your mistakes will for you. Experts agree that for many people the first million dollars you make is the hardest. Once you've learned what it is like to make that kind of money, you'll have an easier time of it going forward—even if you've suffered setbacks along the way, which by the way, most financially successful people have experienced. Stock market losses in the past several years forced many people back into the work force unwillingly. The recent recession has been a wake-up call for many. For others, this turned into a blessing.

DISCOVERING YOUR OWN SECOND ACT

Your next act can be the most exciting and financially rewarding of your life if you are willing to embrace it. If you are one of those talented individuals who have been coasting for a while, open yourself to Your Next Big Thing. Quite often these opportunities are just waiting to fall into your lap if you are open to them and willing to make the changes you know you need to make. Have you developed an expertise that has value in the marketplace? Is there an idea that you are passionate about pursuing? Have you created a product, service, or idea that you can package and sell? You can utilize your past experience to generate additional capital for your future and have more fun than ever during the process.

Centenarian Secret
What's Your Soul Purpose?
Garrett Gunderson, New York Times Bestselling Author of *Killing Sacred Cows*, and founder of Freedom FastTrack, helps individuals and particularly professionals attract more money into their lives. Do you have an expertise, passion or a hobby that you can turn into income? When your work becomes playful, you get an extra bonus in both fun and profit. This is one place where you will generate money through your 100 Year Lifestyle. Visit Garrett's website www.freedomfasttrack.com and YouTube channel www.youtube.com/user/freedomfasttrack for inspiring and motivational information and videos.

Put yourself in position to win and go to work. Be excited about the progress you make, every step of the way. Also, be open to third acts.

For many people, these additional acts are rebirths. You get to start fresh with decades of experience. This is the opportunity of The 100 Year Lifestyle. The opportunities for talented, experienced, motivated, results-oriented people will continue to grow regardless of your age. If you are willing to contribute, truly contribute and not just look for a place to hang your hat and bide your time, you will write your own ticket in any market.

Living The 100 Year Lifestyle: Financial Philosophy

Sir Richard Branson said in a recent Forbes Magazine interview, "I could of course have retired and concentrated my energies on learning how to paint watercolors or how to beat my mum at golf. It wasn't and still isn't in my nature to do so. People asked me, 'Why don't you have some fun now?' but they were missing the point. As far as I was concerned, this was fun. Fun is at the core of the way I like to do business, and it has been key to everything I've done from the outset."

- There is an abundance of money in the world.
- Do what you love.
- Create value for others.
- Create value in the world.
- Package this value in a business.
- Tithe by contributing money to make a difference for others.
- The money will follow.

If you want to achieve abundance throughout your extended life you must do A*Bun*Dance and begin having more fun than ever in your work. What a great way to generate more income as you grow financially free in your extended life.

CREATING YOUR 100 YEAR BALANCE SHEET AND INCOME STATEMENT

The more you invest in yourself, the more freedom and choices you will have. At some stage in your life, you really want to be able to wake up and say, "I want to," rather than, "I have to"—the creativity that comes out of that is exciting. But here is the idea that I really want to get across: It is never too late to start! If you begin thinking this way now, you will attract more abundance right away, regardless of your current age.

This is not just about earning money. It is really about feeling useful and using your talents and abilities to make a difference. The money will be a bonus.

Look at your current personal balance sheet and use it as a tool to gauge where you are on the pathway to financing your 100 Year Lifestyle. What are your current assets? Where is your money allocated? What changes do you need to make to begin to allocate the assets on your balance sheet to increase your cash flow and improve your quality of life as you age?

Your balance sheet represents a snapshot of your financial position and the income streams you will have for the future. What do you want yours to look like during the different stages of life as you age? Meet with your financial advisor and commit to the changes necessary to reach your goals.

- Are you investing in yourself enough to reach your goals?
- Are you investing in things that have meaning for you?
- Do you want to change the way you are allocating your assets or are you happy with your plan?
- Do you have confidence in your plan? Will it meet your needs over your entire life?

I was talking to a doctor who had been running a very successful practice for over 30 years. He was feeling lost and scattered at this stage in his life. When I invited him to do this exercise, he realized that he had real estate investments that were not doing anything for him. He also had flat stocks, mutual funds, and he was funneling his extra income into areas that didn't matter to him anymore and that were underperforming.

He was still working a plan that he had set in place 20 years ago when his values were different and his goals were different. Back when he set those goals for his future, they were exactly what he wanted. Revisiting his goals based on The 100 Year Lifestyle, he realized that his current plan was no longer a plan for his future, but a plan for his past. Not only that, but the world has changed drastically over those 20 years. No wonder he was going backwards.

When I invited him to revisit his goals and meet with his financial advisor to discuss how he could redistribute his assets to finance his current vision for his 100 Year Lifestyle, he began to get excited and inspired. He began to see that if he refocused his financial energy and personal energy toward his passions, he could change things quickly. He sold his property for a nice profit and invested in the mountain retreat he had been wanting for a long time. He took the extra money that was left over and reallocated those assets to meet his current and future goals. He reinvested in his business and brought it up to speed.

In another recent conversation with a different client who was very successful, he began telling me that he was very stressed about money. I couldn't understand it because this doctor had a tremendous income. I asked him to send me over a copy of his balance sheet so I could see where he was allocating his money. After 11 years in practice he had a net worth of approximately $1,800,000. His problem was that he had only around $35,000 in liquid assets. He was taking all of his money and putting it into land. This was going to be a great long-term investment for him; however, he was concerned about the stress that the lack of easy access to cash was causing. For him, it was a matter of finding a dollar amount that would make him feel secure, and reaching that goal before he bought any more land. The sigh of relief I could feel over the phone was huge. I suggested that he talk with his financial advisor and lay out a plan for his 100 Year Lifestyle that would give him the focus and balance he was looking for, and I recommend that you do the same.

Create a balance sheet and income statement that you want to work toward. What types of assets do you want to have—stocks, bonds, commercial real estate, a business, or residential real estate? Do you want to change the way your money works for you to help finance your extended life?

Live Long and Strong: 100 Year Balance Sheet

Create Three Balance Sheets: Title them Current Balance, Desired Balance in 10 Years, and Desired 100 Year Balance. List the following on each Balance Sheet:

Assets

Checking

Money Market

Mutual Funds

Real Estate

Businesses

Miscellaneous

Liabilities

Mortgage

Credit Cards

Leases

Once you decide how you want your 100 Year Balance Sheet and Income Statement to look, you can customize your 100 Year Lifestyle to reach your goals. These statements will give you a path that is filled with passion and financial abundance.

Your financial health will help to remove the stress associated with your potential longevity and get you more excited than ever about your future. When you have confidence in your financial plan you will feel younger, more energetic, and even healthier than you did 10 years ago, especially if you have been following the principles of The 100 Year Lifestyle. Some people spend the first 50 years of their life destroying their health to accumulate wealth, and then they spend the second phase of their life spending their wealth to get their health back. This is the recipe for a 60-year or 70-year lifestyle that you should avoid. There are myriad ways to finance your sensational century. Knowing that you have more time than you ever thought to reach your goals will enable you to achieve financial abundance and keep your health without compromising one for the other.

LIVE LONG AND STRONG
List the talents, skills, and experiences you have accumulated that have value in the marketplace that you would love to utilize to finance your 100 Year Lifestyle:

Talent   Value

1. _____   _____
2. _____   _____
3. _____   _____
4. _____   _____
5. _____   _____

Obviously, the best situation is to start investing in yourself today. Start using your Prep Time to think through business ideas that can finance your fun and exciting 100 Year Lifestyle. The ideal situation is one that gives you the freedom to pursue your interests and the money you need to make them happen. If you follow the Quality Time Living model, you can build so much Play Time into your life, while generating money doing what you love during Prime Time, that you won't feel the need to fully retire. As NY Times bestselling author Garrett Gunderson suggests, "Find your Soul Purpose and commit to it." Some people have turned to real estate to generate income. Your business investments can provide income as well. Many other ideas for generating income may come your way. Be open to the opportunities. Of course, there can be a lot of hard work and some risk involved in this, and I'm not in favor of one strategy or another. You've got to do your homework during your Prep Time and think through your plans thoroughly. I simply want to open your mind to the possibilities and help you identify some opportunities that you may not have considered before.

Financial software programs can help you visualize your life financially. Banks are now offering online resources. Not only can you use them to pay your bills and balance your checkbook, but if you set them up properly, you can also use them to view your balance sheet and income with a click of a button. You can see how your financial life has changed from one year to the next, and you can also use them to paint a picture for the future. Always remember to set goals to finance your 100 Year Lifestyle and use Quality Time Living as a means to reach those goals. Your financial health will enable you to contribute to your family and the world and pave the way for a living legacy that you can enjoy while you are here, and not just after you are gone.

USING YOUR MONEY TO MAKE A DIFFERENCE

Giving back to society is important because it is the right thing to do and it gives your money a purpose. One of my mentors told me that the hole that you give through will determine the size of the hole you receive through. Giving of your time and money is also crucial to your ongoing financial abundance.

One way to give is to tithe, donating a percentage of your income to your favorite causes. You can also stimulate creativity through giving. Ask yourself if there is a cause that you want to raise money for. Brainstorm what you can do with your passion and talents to create a business that generates residual income for your favorite charity, in combination with financing your ideal 100 Year Lifestyle. Mark Victor Hansen, another mentor of mine, has mastered this model and teaches it in his book *Cracking the Millionaire Code* and *One Minute Millionaire*. The amount of money we can all raise when we combine our heartfelt passions, talents, and our extended lives can solve many of the problems in the world. Let's accept this challenge while we also live our dreams, both at the same time.

There are so many resources available to you to make financing your 100 Year Lifestyle more exciting and abundant than you've ever dreamed. Embrace this opportunity with passion as you get ready to live your legacy in the next chapter and truly impact the world.

THE 100 YEAR LIFESTYLE
ACTION PLAN FOR LASTING CHANGE

1. Get excited about the financial opportunity of your 100 Year Lifestyle. Look around and begin to take notice of the resources and experiences you have accumulated and how you can capitalize on them now to create capital for your future.

2. Start investing in yourself. Stop wasting money now. If you have not yet implemented these basics, don't procrastinate another second.

3. Fill in your 100 Year balance sheet based on how it looks today. Decide how you want it to look in ten years and list the five immediate action steps that you know you need to take to reach your goals.

4. Meet with your financial adviser, accountant, estate planner, and insurance agent. Review your financial plan and income opportunities, and make the appropriate changes that will help you secure and finance your 100 Year Lifestyle.

5. Prioritize your own self-care and health care and invest in them. Having the money isn't nearly as much fun if you don't have the health to enjoy it.

6. Check your credit score and credit report. Take the appropriate action steps to clean up any errors.

PART 9

Living Your Legacy for the Rest of Your Life

Imagine a world full of difference makers.

CHAPTER 20

WHY WAIT UNTIL YOU ARE GONE?

The generations before us regarded legacies as something they left behind. But thanks to the fact that we are living longer, we have the opportunity to create legacies while we are still alive. And not just for a few brief years—but for 40, 50 years or more, you will be able to enjoy, shape, and mold your legacy for decades. This concept is important for you, and it is also important to our world as we grapple with the reality that people are living decades longer than expected.

The fact is, you are already creating a legacy every day. How you work, play, and spend time with your family are part of your legacy. The commitment that you have to your community and to raising your children or grandchildren all shape your legacy. But there is another type of legacy—the kind you leave to generations of people that you will never know.

Dr. Ernie Landi, a chiropractor in Chestnut Ridge, New York, is doing just that. Thirty-five years ago, Dr. Landi had a 15-year-old patient walk into his office with excruciating back pain that radiated around to the front of his chest. With every breath, this husky, passionate football player would double over in agony. He had already been to the emergency room and been prescribed medication for the pain. The next day he had gone to an orthopedic surgeon and was prescribed some additional drugs.

Dr. Landi could sense the pain this young man was experiencing from both the injury and his inability to play and help his team win. After a thorough chiropractic examination, Dr. Landi explained the spinal injury he had sustained, called a vertebral subluxation, then adjusted the young athlete—me. I felt immediate relief and went on to play football that afternoon without any pain.

Living The 100 Year Lifestyle: You Never Know How Far Reaching...
In addition to being responsible for over 150 individuals choosing a career in chiropractic, Dr. Ernie Landi has also been honored by his son's choice to follow in his footsteps. Dr. Eric Landi and his wife, Dr. Mallory Becker-Landi, have recently been blessed with twins, Jake and Emma. Because they lived in Atlanta while attending Life University, Dr. Landi was unable to provide his newborn grandchildren the chiropractic care that they needed. Jake's neck was severely subluxated from the way he was positioned in the womb and the trauma of his delivery. The subluxation in his neck caused Jake's neck to be twisted, and the interference to the nervous system was affecting his development, elimination, sleep and ability to nurse. I made a house call to Eric and Mallory's home to adjust the babies. Almost immediately after the adjustment, Jake's head straightened out. He regained full motion in his neck. He slept through the night and his stools were extraordinary. What an honor it was to deliver chiropractic care to my mentor's grandchildren. The impact of Dr. Landi's education, care and lifelong friendship is still growing in influence 35 years later. As B.J. Palmer said, "You never know how far reaching something you say or do today will impact the lives of millions tomorrow."

At the time, Dr. Landi had no idea that I would become an international bestselling author, chiropractor and media personality. He was just doing his job, his passion, every day. He cared for me the same way he cared for every other person that came to see him. Because Dr. Landi was living his legacy every day to the best of his ability, people around the world have been touched by his message through The 100 Year Lifestyle. Still passionately practicing after

40-plus years in Chestnut Ridge, New York, Dr. Landi is living The 100 Year Lifestyle. Through other doctors that he inspired, including me, he is making a difference for people that he doesn't personally know all over the world.

I remember reading recently about Bernie Marcus, one of the Home Depot founders, who had a vision to build hardware stores the size of football fields. Thirty years later, after retiring from Home Depot as a very affluent man, he continues to build and live his legacy. Contributing millions of his own money, he fulfilled another dream by building the Georgia Aquarium in his hometown of Atlanta. His partner at Home Depot is also continuing to live his legacy. Arthur Blank purchased the Atlanta Falcons and turned that team—traditionally a loser—into one of the most exciting teams in the league. We think that people like this are too "big" for us to relate to. Yet, Marcus and Blank were out of work when they were in their forties, prior to starting Home Depot. Today, they continue to find new ways to make exciting contributions to the world and build upon their living legacies.

LIVE LONG AND STRONG
What issues in society are you passionate about that you would like to see changed?
List them here:

_____

_____

_____

_____

Go online and do research on organizations that are involved with solving these challenges. Research these organizations and get involved with the one that most closely connects with your purpose. Or, if the opportunity exists, start one.

Peter Drucker, who had already built an incredible living legacy during his 95 years, completed a book entitled *The Daily Drucker: 366 Days of Insight and Motivation for Getting the Right Things Done,* just before his recent passing. His numerous books have changed the way people do business worldwide. In an article in *USA Today,* Drucker said that at age 95 he was reinventing himself. "What needs to be done now?" He often asked himself this question. He would end up with a new action plan, which he would initiate after asking, "What are the priorities?" He lived his legacy as well as left his legacy to the world.

Why not choose your legacy now so that you have the time to optimize your impact and enjoy the results?

You can move mountains if you just have these two things in your corner: passion and purpose. Find your passion and your purpose and great things will naturally start to come your way.

WHAT WOULD YOU LIKE TO SEE IN YOUR LIFETIME?

What are you deeply passionate about? Do you want to build a building for your church or synagogue? Do you want to be involved in preventing disease or poverty? Do you want to build a company, which favorably impacts the world? Do you want to travel the world with your family? Do you want to write, teach a class, learn a skill, create art, or write music? It's your legacy; what do you want it to be?

At this stage of the game, what do you have to lose? Speak your mind. Get involved. Be a little outrageous. Rather than dwelling on past successes or failures, choose the next phase of the game. Look back and reflect with gratitude and appreciation and remain purposeful, driven, and motivated by Your Next Big Thing.

LEADERSHIP AND THE 100 YEAR LIFESTYLE

How effective you are at living your legacy will be determined by your leadership abilities. There is a Leadership Ladder of The 100 Year Lifestyle with four rungs that must be developed for your living legacy to thrive. These are:

1. Personal Leadership
2. Professional Leadership
3. Community Leadership
4. Global Leadership

As you climb The Leadership Ladder, your quality of life and your legacy will improve dramatically and the impact that you have on the planet will be extraordinary.

PERSONAL LEADERSHIP

Over the course of your 100 years, you're going to come in contact with thousands and thousands of people. By now, I'm sure you've learned that every one of these people has an opinion about what is the right thing for you. Everyone wants to tell you what you should be doing, what you should eat, and what is best for your life. At some point, you're going to have to decide to lead yourself. Personal Leadership is about trusting yourself and directing yourself, throughout your life, so that you can fulfill your destiny and reach the potential you were created to achieve.

Choose your Dominant Energy Pattern to be about your human potential. Choose the attitude that attracts health, happiness, and success for a lifetime; create your personal Renewal Recipe and follow it; discipline yourself to follow through on what you know is right for you. Lead yourself with Quality Time Living, finance your 100 Year Lifestyle, and embrace the Health Care Hierarchy for the quality of life you desire and deserve. Embrace the Personal Leadership that is necessary for you to reach your goals and use your talents and abilities to the fullest. Nobody can truly lead you except *you*.

Leading Generations To Healthier Lifestyle Choices

Contributed by Ashley Hecht, C.A. at Koca Chiropractic

In my position as a Chiropractic Assistant, I am privileged to witness healthy transitions I never thought possible. I've learned from Dr. Lyle Koca and the doctors in our office that lives can be changed and transformed. Kids become healthy, athletes are able to compete at their highest ability, and elderly patients don't show the same signs of suffering that most aging people show. The highlight is the families that come in together to see us and the parents who head those households. The changes are amazing and the entire family benefits.

One of our patients, Connie, was living a stress-filled, busy life as a mother and grandmother while employed full-time, plus caring for out-of-town rental properties. She was worn out! Like many people, she was living on quick meals and caffeine and physically feeling the effects of her hectic lifestyle.

Although skeptical at first, Connie noticed a significant difference in how she felt shortly after she started care. Less headaches, more energy, and less pain were enough for Connie to quickly realize she had discovered a better way of living. She was so excited and interested in her transformation that she began to question why everyone did not utilize chiropractic care as a main source of healthcare. She encouraged her family to come in and get checked. They loved it! Now, a year later, Connie's friends, children and grandchildren are experiencing its benefits. One of Connie's granddaughters who had a long list of ear infections, antibiotics, and tubes has been medication free since she started care.

I am a big believer that if mom is healthy, the family is healthier. When we, as parents, put ourselves last our health falters and everyone in our family suffers. The 100 Year Lifestyle and chiropractic principles are the way to achieve a healthy lifestyle for ourselves and our families. Connie has come to see this first-hand and has gone out and shared this with the community. Connie is striving to live to 100 and beyond and see her family achieve this as well. The world needs more women like her to lead others and spread the message.

PROFESSIONAL LEADERSHIP

As you build your Personal Leadership skills and test them out in the world, you'll probably have the opportunity to develop your Professional Leadership. This comes with experience and is achieved by creating results in your career. But how will you know if you are on the right track? How will you know if people respect you? How will you know if you are effective? It's simple. Look behind you and ask: "Who is following me?"

Do you remember the childhood game Follow the Leader? The leader would perform an action, and everyone else would follow accordingly. In life, you can gauge your ability to lead by looking back to see who is following you. You may turn around and see that nobody is following you. This is a wake-up call. Personal Leadership is about embracing the characteristics that make people want to follow you. Professional Leadership is how you apply these qualities in your career.

You may look behind you and see destructive people following you. Do you have a group of alcoholics who follow you to a bar every night? Are you leading people to a new credit card with the latest point system, while you go further and further into the hole? This is a great way to learn your level of leadership.

On the other hand, you may look behind you and find that other leaders are now following you. Congratulations. You're on your way. This is a very concrete indicator that you have become effective at what you do. As we discussed throughout this book, have patience and expect some time for you to develop. Rome wasn't built in a day. Your life and legacy won't be either. This goes back to the Titration Principle we spoke about earlier. The concept of The 100 Year Lifestyle should give you a new, fresh, and exciting take on leadership. You have time to raise a family, earn a living, invest in yourself and your future and focus on issues in your world that you care about. The better you get at managing the things that you love, the more good things you will attract. Before you know it, you will become a leader in your professional life, which comes with an exciting array of benefits for you to enjoy over your lifetime.

COMMUNITY LEADERSHIP

Community Leadership has to do with making a difference in your immediate world. This may be your neighborhood, a church, synagogue, athletic community, cultural community, or a community that is connected to one of your hobbies. Assuming a leadership role in the community will keep you growing, connected, involved, and inspired over the course of your 100 years. Community Leadership will give you a sense of purpose and connect you to the greater good. Use your skills in the community to make a difference.

Every organization is looking for people who care about their cause and who are willing to get involved. Pick a cause you are passionate about and be a difference maker by offering your time and talents. The people you read about in the newspapers and see on television who seem to be extraordinary people are usually just ordinary people who decided to step up to the plate.

The opportunities are everywhere.

GLOBAL LEADERSHIP

Global Leadership is about changing the world. By climbing the Leadership Ladder yourself, and then spreading the word to everyone you know, one titration drop at a time, this crazy world will change. Isn't that exciting?

What would happen if we all embraced The 100 Year Lifestyle and the reality of our extended life span and used our unique and cumulative talents in this way? This commitment to leadership on a personal, professional, and community level would absolutely change the world. When I think about how extended life spans are going to affect my children, my grandchildren, and my great-grandchildren, I think about the kind of world that they will inherit from us. And sometimes I worry. I don't ever want them to be afraid to go to school because of violence. I don't want them to fear being attacked there, or anywhere else for that matter. I don't ever want them to find themselves in situations where they may be tempted to try dangerous drugs. I worry about whether they will be impacted by intolerance, hatred, and bigotry. And I worry about a "world divided," which will only produce terror and isolationism.

By choosing a cause that you are passionate about and working to make a difference, you will be changing the globe by impacting your piece of it. What's so great is that we have an opportunity to use our extended lives to make the world a much better place. Knowing that we have more time on the planet than we ever thought we would, we might actually be able to solve some important problems. Think globally and act locally for a lifetime, and you will be exercising Global Leadership.

LIVE LONG AND STRONG
It's time for you to climb the Leadership Ladder. Under each rung of the ladder below, list three actions or characteristics you can implement immediately that would make you more passionate about your life and that would make you more of the kind of person that other people want to follow.
Personal leadership:

_____
_____
_____

Professional leadership:

_____
_____
_____

Community leadership:

_____
_____
_____

Global leadership:

_____
_____
_____

MAINTAINING LASTING PURPOSE, DRIVE, AND MOTIVATION

Compare the stories you have read in this book to the one about Max, the man I introduced you to early on. Do you remember Max? He was the elderly gentleman who died crippled, broke and alone. Max was 100 years old when he died, and I don't know why he was so crippled, broke, or so alone in the world. Maybe he was predisposed to holding people at arm's length. Maybe he valued the wrong things in life. Maybe he experienced some losses in his life from which he was never able to recover. But my thoughts about Max inspired me to write this book. Max was a very sweet man and his life touched me.

I want you to enjoy an incredible quality of life for your entire life. This means trusting your Innate Intelligence and making conscious choices every day—from now to 80, 90, 100 and beyond.

If you:
- Are working all the time and sacrificing your important relationships, stop.
- Are financially just living for today and aren't investing in your future, stop.
- Aren't taking care of your body, stop.
- Think you'll never find love again following a painful divorce or premature death of your partner, stop.
- Think you are done contributing to the world by the time you reach "retirement," stop.
- Are busy trying to control other people or are allowing others to control you, stop.
- Are angry about the past, stop.
- Are playing the victim, stop.

You deserve to have it all and experience life to the fullest, and you will have plenty of time to make it happen. Although it might be a little scary starting over at your stage of life, start over anyway and cultivate courage and energy-enhancing attitudes that become a way of life and part of your new human potential pattern.

When you focus your life on things that are meaningful to you, you will have a lasting drive. Being passionate about your life is the key to mastering your life. Commit to things greater than yourself.

Don't worry about what you can't change. You'll discover that messy details in your life start to right themselves on their own as you commit and recommit yourself every day. You'll attract answers. Ruminating is the surest way to stay stuck.

Recently, *USA Today Weekend* reported that a Dutch psychologist tried to figure out what separated chess masters from chess grand masters. He subjected groups of each to a battery of tests, including IQ, memory, and spatial reasoning. He found no testing difference between them. The only difference was that grand masters simply loved chess more. They had more passion and commitment to the game of chess.

Your purpose is your choice. There are so many ways you can make a difference in the world with your unique talents and abilities. The world is waiting for you to step up to the plate. Start climbing that ladder and enjoy the journey every step of the way.

CHAPTER 21

FROM GENERATION TO GENERATION—FOR 100 YEARS AND BEYOND

When my children were in grade school they had to do a family tree project. I remember teaching them a little about my grandparents. But in reality, I hardly knew them. They passed away when I was relatively young. My kids also asked me about my great-grandparents. I shared a few details about them, but not too much. A few facts had been passed down. But otherwise, my mind was pretty much a blank slate. I basically knew nothing about them. They lived for decades and I'm sure shared many of my same joys and struggles. My kids' lesson made me wonder at the time about their lives. What were they like? What motivated them? What were there likes and dislikes? It would have been great to get to know them better.

Our longevity may be blessed with the opportunity to know many future generations of our family including great grandchildren and great, great grandchildren. I remember watching my Papa Hy get on the floor and play passionately with his great-grandchildren when they were small, even when he was 100 years old. Their youthful exuberance made him feel younger. He fed off of it. He gave back to them through his playfulness and wisdom. The energy exchange was intense for everyone. Since his passing at 100 years old and nine months, we all have been blessed with memories of him. He got to

100 with no knowledge or thought that he would live that long. He got there by accident.

We are the first generation in history that is getting the advance notice that our parents and grandparents never received that we will probably live longer than we ever thought. What will you do with this information? You and I have the opportunity to get there in style and with purpose. Let's make our time really matter.

> **Centenarian Secret**
> We all have a history. I don't want yours and you don't want mine. What's more important than your history is your commitment.

ANTI-AGING AND ACTIVISM

Get involved and select your cause. Whether it's working for your church or synagogue, the environment, children, women's rights, poverty, homelessness, or AIDS prevention, pick something that matters to you and get involved. Make a difference in your own little piece of the world. Find a few causes close to home and start making an impact. Don't assume your voice is of no consequence. Don't curse the direction in which the world is moving. Put your paddle in the water and start rowing.

Your voice absolutely does matter. Several years ago I was flying back from speaking at a seminar. My neighbor on the plane was a woman who was feeling suppressed in her marriage and did not feel free to express her voice in her marriage, or anywhere else for that matter. As she tried to talk about it, her voice kept getting weaker, as if her throat were closing up. I asked her to shift her posture to a confident position while she wiped the negativity away by gently and artistically waving her fingers across her throat, and then tossing the pain aside. She did it. Instantly her voice got stronger. I suggested that she sit or stand confidently and repeat this motion each time she wants to express herself and she feels her voice locking up. She followed my suggestion and today she is working in a new job selling a computer software program, and through her job she has to give one-hour sales presentations to potential customers. She found her voice all right, and you should find yours. You will love finding your voice and when you do, it will change your life forever.

Respect the generational shifts. Learn about societal changes and why they are taking place. Be a good listener and learn as much as you can while you also respect your own experiences. Know that you bring something unique to the table. Find a way to be heard. Now, I understand that sometimes the world can look or feel like an awfully big place. We can feel powerless. But by getting involved in the causes that matter to you, the world will feel much more like an extended community. You will become part of something bigger. You will experience the joy of making a positive contribution in your corner of the world. An important part of aging well is to always keep a sense of purpose. Always.

Living The 100 Year Lifestyle: Mary Lou Ciulla

Mary Lou Ciulla, lost her husband, Frank, in a terrorist attack on December 21, 1988. He was a passenger on Pan Am flight 103, which exploded over Lockerbie, Scotland.

"I experienced a broad spectrum of emotions the day I found out my husband died. I was just in shock. There was no anger, initially. There was, however, a tremendous longing to have been with him. I felt profound sadness that he was alone that day—so far from home and in the company of strangers—when he was murdered. He was a brilliant, kind, and compassionate man. And now he was gone. Forever.

I still had three kids to look after. I soon recognized that I would have to lead them through this. If I came through this okay, they would be okay. But we had all been traumatized. Months went by and we started to resume a routine. A little emotional healing had taken place, which opened me up to a new phase: Anger. I began to feel the fury.

I explained it to my children. I said that I thought my anger was starting to come out, and I needed to focus it on someone or something before it took over. I didn't want to direct it toward my children, my friends, or people who didn't understand. My support system was obviously more important than ever. It was actually through harnessing these powerful emotions that I started to find meaning again. The first step was joining a support group with other Pan Am flight 103 families. We all shared the same experience and understood each other's feelings. We were going through the same grieving process. We didn't have to explain or defend our reactions. Through the process, I began to realize that Frank really wasn't alone that day. He was in the company of good people, with wonderful families back home. My mind was now stepping outside of my loss and was starting to register the bigger picture. This was the beginning of true healing for me.

The Pan Am flight 103 families became an extended community. Valuable friendships were formed that still endure today. And we began to apply what we had learned.

A second milestone came on September 11, 2001. I immediately started a support group for wives who lost husbands that day. I partnered with a dear friend who lost her husband on Pan Am flight 103. We hosted weekly support group meetings in our homes. We supported the widows emotionally and in every way we possibly could. My kids were more concerned about me going back in time, but to be honest, it helped me to help them. They would ask us things like, "Does the pain ever go away?" We were very honest with them; we told them that it doesn't. But we explain how it changes. When this happens, you get a big hole in your stomach—that hole is the person you lost. That person is gone and you can never replace him. But what happens is that you shrink that hole in your stomach with little things the rest of your life. And it fills up again with a lot of little things.

When you see the expression on someone's face change because you have really connected with her and helped her, it's a terrific feeling. I was willing to do that over and over again. Years later, I take great pride in seeing how they have progressed. They are further along that I was after the same amount of time. The key is that they had the proper support, right away.

Currently, I'm also in the process of initiating an ongoing program for Northern New Jersey on traumatic grief—surviving the loss of a loved one to a traumatic death. This program has been highly successful in the southern part of the state and so I held a fundraiser in my husband's memory to raise funds to bring it to northern New Jersey.

Today, I have five grandchildren, I have two great son-in-laws, and my kids are doing well and living full, happy lives. I have many wonderful nieces and nephews. All these things are things my husband can't share with me, but I'm still glad to have them. These are the things that fill you up over the years.

When my husband first died, it was like I wanted to die too. But now I realize I would have missed out on all of this. I believe that I still have a long life ahead of me. I see my aunts and parents living well into their nineties and it's important to me, knowing that I have longevity on my side, to make my life have meaning.

Involvement makes your life matter. It brings healing and joy, versus complacency, and keeps it fun.

You can stay with the same cause for months, years, and decades or you can rotate your time and energy on a project basis. The choice is up to you. The important thing is that you get involved in something bigger than yourself. You will meet new people, make new friends, and you may create new business opportunities. But more than anything, you will bring new meaning to your life. Just be sure to pick causes that really resonate with your soul. Don't simply join a group or volunteer for a blood drive and expect your life to change overnight! In fact, identifying causes that are meaningful to you can take a little soul-searching. The key is to get started and to get involved.

Think about the things that you take notice of during the day— things that may even dismay you. What issues do you talk about with friends, family, and neighbors? For example, you may live in a part of the country that is very scenic and laid-back, and you may fear the encroachment of developers. By all means, get involved. This is not a time to roll over. The world has enough problems as it is, without people destroying its natural beauty. Get passionately involved.

You don't even have to start big. In this case, you could begin by organizing a cleanup day in your neighborhood. Get some neighbors together and just start picking up all the trash. Through this small chore, you will soon find yourself connecting with the earth. You'll see your world a little differently. A friend of mine did this with a group from her neighborhood one weekend. She watched a driver go speeding by and hit a deer. The deer died right at her feet. This particular region contains a large nature preserve being consumed by developers. She told me that when she saw the impact, firsthand, it deepened her desire to preserve the region where she lives.

A few years ago, I chose to put a lot of energy into the nonprofit organization founded by Stedman Graham in 1985 called Athletes Against Drugs. This organization exists to inspire and educate kids on the importance of living healthy, drug-free lives. My kids were teenagers at the time and I wanted to keep them safe, healthy, and drug free. I feel very strongly that there are too many young athletes using drugs—both performance enhancing and street drugs. They think it will help them compete, but they are not considering their ideal 100 Year Lifestyle. They are not thinking long-term and many are simply ignorant about the consequences of their choices. Connecting to this cause kept my passion burning to make a difference in the world. It was exciting. I got to meet great people. I tapped into new avenues of creativity, and I felt a strong sense of purpose because of my commitment. Research organizations like this in your community and get involved.

There are so many ways to get involved and make a difference. Being in service is one of the greatest gifts you can give to the world, and it is also the greatest gift you can give to yourself.

Why wait until you are gone? If you are going to live longer than you ever thought you would, why not make it worthwhile? Give yourself permission to engage in your life in a way that you never have before.

Centenarian Secret

If at any time in your life you've had a burn in your gut to do something, accomplish something, try something, and really express your heartfelt passions, now is the time to do it. The truth is, desire has probably always been with you and will never really go away. It may dim from some challenges. But just like a fire, if you give it a little poke, the flames reignite.

I want to live in a world where people everywhere are making their lives matter. I want my children and their children to experience a world where people are committed to creating meaningful legacies and living passionate lives. Anything is possible when you tap into the depths of your own human potential.

I truly believe that everyone deserves to be healthy and express their full potential—from the time they are born through their last breath of life. The choices we make today will impact our quality of life today and in our future. They will also impact the world, since we are all more intimately connected than ever before. I want to live in a world where this is happening. I would love to experience the beauty of that world for myself, my family, and my future grandchildren, and for you; a world in which people are living their full potential— truly living their ideal 100 Year Lifestyle.

Living The 100 Year Lifestyle: Jacob Plasker

When my son Jacob was born, Lisa and I were proud parents. I had grand visions for his life and believed he was destined for greatness. I couldn't wait to share an incredible life with him. I believed he could live an extraordinary 100 years. When he was born, he had everything in place to be able to do that. Unfortunately, when he was ten months old, he had an accident that caused him to be paralyzed. All the experts told us that he would never walk, talk, or use his right arm. Through a strong belief in the healing powers of the human body, chiropractic care, incredible faith, and a lot of the self-care, health care, and crisis care strategies mentioned through The 100 Year Lifestyle, he has regained his health and is living to his potential. He has an incredible life ahead of him and he has grown into a dynamic, handsome, and quality young man. He is an honors graduate from the University of Georgia's Terry School of Business with a degree in Finance and he just started chiropractic studies at Life University. His healing inspired my passion for human potential to a whole new level. This power to heal, be healthy, live in abundance, and make a difference in the world is in every one of us. It is the essence of The 100 Year Lifestyle.

HERE'S TO US

I would like to end this book with a nod to my wife's grandfather, Hyman Sperling, who turned 100 on December 7, 2006. He and his wife, Henrietta, were married for 60 years. His advice, which has always stayed with me, is brilliant yet simple: "Be true to your loved ones, your friends, and your buddies. Closeness and companionship are all you need." I would like to add one more thing to that: Be true to yourself. Be true to your heart's desire and live with passion. Have you ever noticed that people who live with passion just seem to get better, year after year? That's what The 100 Year Lifestyle is all about: living an incredible life, every day of your life, for 80, 90, 100 years and beyond.

So, here's to us. May we all enjoy and experience a sensational century. I hope to meet you along the way. God bless.

THE 100 YEAR LIFESTYLE
ACTION PLAN FOR LASTING CHANGE

1. Live your legacy every day. Starting with today, make every interaction you have with other people a positive one. Look for the good in each person and stand for your best legacy today.

2. Have gratitude for your past and look to the future with the promise of your ideal 100 Year Lifestyle. What are the changes you know you need to make to live the legacy that resides in your genetic core? What would you like to see in your lifetime? Go for it. If you don't, you probably won't see it. If you do, you surely will.

3. Lead yourself. Nobody is going to do it for you. You know what is right for you. Lead yourself.

4. Develop your professional, community, and global leadership skills. Get involved in your profession and continue to develop your skills. Set goals that will force you to learn the necessary skills you will need to live your ideal 100 Year Lifestyle.

5. Get involved. Get active. Choose a cause that matters to you and commit yourself to making a difference. Let your voice be heard.

6. Embrace your family and multiple generations. Look around you and identify both the younger and older people in your

life that you would like to get to know better. Make a phone call. Get a date on the calendar.

7. Enjoy the journey on your way to a sensational century.

I choose to fail.
I choose to succeed.
I choose to extinguish.
I choose to ignite.
I choose to get by.
I choose to excel.
I choose to follow.
I choose to lead.
I choose to drift.
I choose to commit.
I choose my choices.
I choose my life.

I CHOOSE MY LIFE

By Dr. Eric Plasker

I choose to die.
I choose to live.
I choose to hate.
I choose to love.
I choose to close.
I choose to open.
I choose to cry.
I choose to laugh.
I choose to deny.
I choose to believe.
I choose to ignore.
I choose to hear.
I choose to be right.
I choose to relate.
I choose to scatter.
I choose to focus.
I choose to work.
I choose to play.
I choose to be angry.
I choose to accept.
I choose to despair.
I choose to hope.
I choose to give up.
I choose to persist.
I choose to suffer.
I choose to heal.
I choose to destroy.
I choose to create.